GENIUS YOU

www.thegeniusyou.com

THE GENIUS YOU

written by

MANOJ CHHABLANI

ADHYYAN BOOKS

The Genius You

1st Edition

Publication Date: March 2020

Price: ₹399 | $ 11.99

ISBN: 978-93-88644-65-5

Published by:

Adhyyan Books

Office No. 637,

Opposite Vivanta by Taj,

DDA SFS. Pocket-1, Dwarka,

Sec-22, New Delhi-110077

Website: http://adhyyanbooks.com

E-mail: contact@adhyyanbooks.com

Dedication

I dedicate this book to my late grandparents, for their unparalleled love and values that they've inculcated. They are not alive but they always remains alive in my heart.

About the Author

Mr. Manoj Chhablani is highly influential, Inspiring and impactful individual, known for building high performing teams. His passion for unleashing the potential of individuals and coaching them to perform at their peak has made wonders for several individuals and teams. Personal transformation and personal excellence is an area where he's deeply passionate about and created wonderful result over a period of decade and half as a 'Head of Operations' in 2 technology companies that he's associated with.

When he's not creating magic at work or spending time with his family, he can usually be found enhancing his knowledge by reading a book and that book will more likely be a non-fiction. He can also be seen singing occasionally in family gatherings or watching movies with his family & friends but his hunger to learn strategies on personal excellence never goes off!

Mr. Chhablani, a certified performance coach and Neuro Linguistic Programming (NLP) expert, strongly believes the best investment someone can makes is in themselves. He's obsessed for bringing new ideas to work and transforming HR (Human Resources) to HPR (High Performing Resources). Having a book on personal transformation under his name was one of his dream and eventually it become a reality with this book.

Mr. Chhablani is not a full-time writer but writing non-fiction and sharing his strategies on personal excellence always makes him excited about. 'The Genius you' is his first deliberate attempt to start his journey as an author to influence, inspire and impact you reaching your personal excellence and think, act & live like a 'Genius'. Don't miss a chance to e-connect with him at www.manojchhablani.com

About 'The Genius You'

Message by Author:

Sometimes it just takes one person, one book, one article, one podcast, or just one video to tell you how exceptional, capable and worthy individual you are to live a life you wish to. Let me be that somebody thru this book and let that day be today and that moment be now.

If you feel the moment for positive changes in your life is not now and can be a little later than you are procrastinating to unleash your potential and the more you procrastinate the less time it'll be for you to enjoy the success of performing at your peak. Not just that, if you keep procrastinating, who knows you'll never ever get time to take on to this journey. Don't wait any further, it's now or never, go ahead and choose to be a genius, unleash your potential and perform with your maximum potential. If you're up for this journey to personal excellence than you've wonderful insights in this book ahead to take you to that journey.

Wow! The fact that you're still holding this book in your hand indicates you don't want to wait anymore in transforming your life to next level and that's what takes you in top 5% of the people that are serious about their life and want to do something meaningful. You could have opted to have something entertaining that could have given you the short burst but you choose to read this book and have longer term impact in your life. Congratulations! You deserve a pat on your back!

This books is not just a motivational book like any other self-help book, it's all about personal transformation, and the journey to personal transformation is to execute & move from complexity to simplicity. This book describes all my learnings and experiences that helped me and several others transforming their lives to different level and the same could happen to you as well. I don't claim myself to be a genius yet, but with the continuous guidance of my mentor, I'm already on my way and what is important is, I'm aware about what it takes to be a genius, this awareness is the first step and then comes the execution part (which is most crucial to be successful) is what this book talks about.

The Genius You = Genius Inside + Genius Outside

The roadmap to 'The Genius You' is being 'Genius inside' and 'Genius outside'. This book is the blueprint or roadmap to be a genius, if you follow the map you could identify your true potential and ways on performing with your maximum potential, it guides you on which direction you've to move during your journey to reach to your goals. It doesn't matter which field you're operating into, which stage you are in your personal life, which position you're holding in your organization, or which stage you are in your entrepreneurial journey, following what has been mentioned in this book can bring transformation in your life. I always believe in practicality and what works in real life, this book is not about what we should do and what we shouldn't, it's about what works and what doesn't.

There is no doubt that, all the transformation happens inside out and it's your inner strength that determines how you are approaching to various external factors. This book not just focuses on how you can build your inner strength but also guides you on what external factors to pay attention to in order to excel your performance. There are number of topics covered in this book and each topic can be a separate book in itself but you can treat these as a quick guide of various pre-requisites to maximize your performance. If you read this book completely and follow the way it's expected than you will get introduced to new version of you who can conquer anything in this world. This book also shares a buffet of winning strategies and success methods that works in practical life and already being used by several billionaires that change their lives. Last but not the least you'll find ways on how to change negative beliefs, have growth mindset and reprogram your subconscious mind and be a winner by taking massive actions. The content, ideas and strategies shared in this book won't make any difference unless you execute them and live with them in your daily life.

Having this book in your hand shows the fire in your belly and I urge you not to let this fire cool off until you accomplish what you wish to. I don't know which age group you're falling into but I'll urge you not to wait anymore and start acting now. Unstuck yourself, roar like a lion, reinvent the new you and join this exciting journey ahead! You've a wonderful opportunity to leave a legacy but this will happen if you take action. I don't want you to get late and regret few years from now on why you haven't taken this journey earlier! Act now!

"There is no perfect moment, you've to take the moment and make it perfect"

Acknowledgements

For not full time writers like myself, this book is a big accomplishment but for this dream to become a reality several others have given me the strength and contributed directly-indirectly to make this happen. It is with deep gratitude that I acknowledge and thank everyone for their contribution.

To start with, thanks to my parents for the upbringing, blessings, continued support & confidence in my capabilities that make me believe from 'Can I' to 'I can' and this book is the result of my strong belief that says 'I Can'.

Thanks to my wife, Bhaveshi and my son Prayansh to continue to push me and sacrificing the personal family time while I'm writing during late night and early morning. Without your support this book wouldn't have been possible.

Thanks to my mentors, Mr. Bhupendra Singh Rathore and Arfeen Khan for igniting me and guiding me to be an author. Your mentorship has brought incredible changes to my life. You have been the true inspiration for me to touch any heights that I can think of.

Thanks to my brothers Ramesh & Vinod, all my cousins and other family members, several mastermind group, BNI group, IMA members, all my teachers during my educational journey, and all the friends in my social circle for the real life lessons to deal with various situation in the day to day life. I'm blessed to count you all as my well-wishers.

Special thanks to real differentiators in my life Mr. K.L. Mamnani, Manish Mamnani and Parag Mamnani for believing in me and mentoring me over the years. Thanks to all the colleagues at Gate6 and Webgility office for my work related education over the years. Can't forget to thank the office boys for getting me a cup of coffee to energize me at work.

Thanks to all the books, Articles, Blogs, Videos, podcasts for the learnings and motivation.

Finally, I thank god for giving me the strength, resources, environment, culture and real life situations that is allowing me to do what I love that serves several others.

Thank you everyone, you all contributed to all good things that brought me here so far and I'm blessed to count you all in my life.

Index

Chapter 1

WHY GENIUS?

"It's not okay to be okay."

If you feel, being genius or successful is difficult, look at the life of people who are not successful and see how difficult their life is. If you think to become a genius, a lot of efforts are required then look at the life of people that are not genius and how mediocre their life is. Being genius initially takes some effort but the benefits that you are going to reap for the rest of your life are really unbelievable.

Why to live a mediocre life when you can live like a rockstar? God has not sent us in this world to only work, eat and sleep. We have been given this beautiful life to make an impact, to do something significant and positive that people remember even after we are not alive, to do something meaningful that gives us satisfaction, and to achieve the heights that we are capable of.

You have only one life to make an impact in this entire world and you can't allow your potential to go waste in the areas that don't fetch any value. You can't leave your luck to decide your success. Being mediocre is not our maximum potential, our potential is limitless and not utilizing our true potential is not justifiable with the purpose we have been sent for in this world by the Almighty God. Don't ask yourself, "Why Genius", ask yourself "Why not Genius?"

It's not mandatory to have a rich or successful uncle in order to be rich or successful. It's your internal and external preparation which anybody can have if they decide to do so and put their efforts. It's just a matter of following simple rules on a regular basis.

I know the reason why you are holding this book and still reading, this shows you want to perform up to your potential and if you feel this is not the right time, ask yourself one more question, "Why not now?" The early you start, the better and faster are the chances for you to trek to the peak.

"Mediocrity will never do. You are capable of something better."

- Gordon B. Hinckley

What does it take to be a genius?

People who are geniuses out there, killing it in life, are not luckier than most. They don't believe in 'luck', they feel they are the captain of their ship and the master of their destiny. They believe in their talent, efforts and their beliefs. They know success is not just random or a co-incidence. They just do things that others are not willing to do:

§ They have passion and purpose in life, which most people don't have.

§ They stretch their efforts a little further each day.

§ They use their time in a way most people won't do.

§ They know their 'Why', which most people don't know.

§ They have a set of habits that most people don't have.

§ They treat challenges and obstacles as opportunities which most people won't do.

In short, they continue to give their best every single day and are passionate about their goal to keep moving forward with motivation.

Being a genius one single day, one single week or one single month will not bring the transformation that we are looking for.

It's about being a genius every single day and continuing with the same for the rest of the life. This requires a complete change and that change is possible by doing simple things but most of us believe in complexity and we feel people who are geniuses belong to a different category. However, they all are same like any mediocre. The only difference is they are clear about their goal and they are ready to endeavor whatever it takes to chase their goal. If we want to be among the top 5% of the people, we have to act like the top 5% of people.

So, are you ready to be a genius? If not, great news... you don't have to read this book any further. But if you are ready to board the journey to be a genius, you are on a treat. Remember this quote by Robin Sharma;

"All changes are hardest in the beginning, messy in the middle and gorgeous in the end."

What got you here, won't get you where you want to be

Evaluate your personal and professional life and analyze the result that you have got so far. Do you feel you are able to perform with your true potential? Do you feel you could have done much better? I'll keep repeating over and again that your potential is limitless, the sky is the limit for you. Ask yourself, "Have I reached my potential so far?"

If you feel you have not lived to your potential, think about why you have not been able to accomplish what you are capable of. What has stopped you so far? Are you afraid of taking massive actions? My guess is either you miss some inner fire that holds you back, you don't have the blueprint of success or you are taking mediocre actions that are only drifting you to mediocrity. Do these sounds familiar? Well, you can't just do random things and expect a miracle to happen in life.

If you want to be a genius, want to be successful or if you want to be among the top 5% achievers, you have to stop doing things that bottom 95% people are doing. You must start focusing on what top 5% achievers are doing. It's your choice, but yes, if you choose to be among the top 5% then you have to think, act and execute in an entirely different way. And when you do that it's becomes a game-changer.

The core lies in your thinking and belief system. If you start thinking and believing like successful people, your confidence and commitment entirely soar to a different level. That's how you don't crumble when the going gets rough.

If you want to be successful, you have to consistently model the strategies and habits of successful people, make the best use of time by prioritizing the most critical items, have clear goals, conquer your fear and take consistent action.

Your energy and motivation play a big role in this entire journey. Surround yourself with the close group of high-performers to continue fueling yourself with the required motivation. Stay energetic for the same vibration to be transported to others.

Remember, if you want to get something you have never got, you have to do something that you have never done. Average efforts bring average results, massive actions bring massive transformation. Go ahead! Unleash the genius within, you are born to be a winner, come out of the mediocrity and unleash the **new you.** The whole world is waiting for you to make an impact but the only question is, Are you ready? Say, Yes! And move on.

"The Harvest you reaped today was the result of your seed you planted yesterday. If you didn't like what you got, plant better seeds for tomorrow"

- Elle Sommer

Chapter 2

ACTIVATE YOUR POTENTIAL

"Untapped potential is the difference between where a person is now and where he or she can be."

- Bo Bennett

Have you ever played a video game beyond level 4?

Have you ever played a video game? The whole idea of a video game is to move up to another level, then another level and as the level goes higher, the game gets tougher but we also become tougher. Can you imagine a video game that has 10 levels and never being able to pass level 4? What is crazy is that most people live their life like that and are never able to pass level 4. And what's funnier is, they enjoy playing level 1-3 over and again...Why? Because when they play level 1-3, they enjoy the sweet taste of success, whereas level 4 and above give them the bitter feeling of failure. So, they never try to be in that zone and don't even try for that. Think about it; why do you restrict yourself to level 4? What is your potential is? What are you capable of?

Are you an eagle or a pigeon?

There are two types of people, Eagles or Pigeons. When a pigeon wants something to eat, it waits on the ground in the park for some old lady to throw crumbs or you will see pigeons lurking by fighting over scraps. They have to wait for someone to throw some discards and they only get what's left for them.

On the other hand, when an Eagle wants to eat something, it goes to the top of a mountain, soars down and plucks a fish twice its size out of the water or grabs another bird out in the sky and starts eating it in the mid-flight. Instead of waiting in the wings for somebody to throw something on the ground, it rather takes the action flight and seizes its treat. It doesn't just hope that it can find something, it goes out and gets what it wants.

What about you? Are you waiting for an opportunity to knock your door? Or you are waiting for the right moment? Don't wait for the right moment or an opportunity, take the moment and make it perfect!

Unleash your potential

Each individual has tremendous amount of potential, and they can do much more than what they can think of, but for majority of them, their potential is either dormant or unutilized. Most of them have not been able to discover what their true potential is because like a video game, they don't even try for level 4 and above. They just wait like a pigeon that keeps them at bay from not even identifying their true capacity.

Identifying your peak potential can be one of the greatest discoveries of your life. You can't imagine how your life can be transformed when the potential is discovered, nurtured and properly utilize in the best possible way.

Have you ever thought about what your potential is? And what is the level you are currently operating your life at? Probably not. And if you determine your true potential with your current level of performance, then you have to rethink about it because several times we are not been able to perform to our true potential for a variety of reasons which we will be covering here.

Does everyone have potential? How to discover the true potential? How to identify your peak-potential and get into action mode for the outcome that you deserve?

Centric thought:

"Potential is a priceless treasure, like gold. All of us have gold hidden within, but we have to dig to get it out."

- Joyce Meyer

Pledge: I have a tremendous amount of potential, I will do whatever it takes to discover it, nurture it and utilize it in the best possible way and leave a legacy.

Does everyone have Potential?

One of the Greek philosophers spoke about 'entelechy' which means the potentiality that is there within every living being, within us, within every aspect of nature. In fact, the potentiality of the acorn is to become a great oak tree. The acorn, when activated, cannot become an orange tree. It can only become a great oak tree; it's wired that way. And each one of us is wired in the same way for greatness.

Metaphysics, the role of quantum physics and quantum mechanics, also say that anything we put our focus on repeatedly with action and emotion will manifest itself. Greatness is within us.

There are thousands of books written about people who have achieved greatness yet started from a humble beginning. Within us, each and every one of us has the potential for greatness, brilliance and unique talent to fill a very specific need in the world. We have been sent by God while being inherited with a wonderful gift, this gift is our talent . All we have to do is identify that gift, nurture it and employ it to the best use.

No matter what people say, each one of us has a tremendous amount of potential. Several times, we ignore that fact and start believing what other people tell us, which is the prime reason for us not to discover our true potential. Hence, we continue with what we have been forced to believe about ourselves.

We have not been sent by God for a mediocre life. There is a much better purpose for which we have been sent on this earth. And the Gift that we are born with, what lies inside us is our true potential, this is what can help us fulfill that purpose.

All we have to do is identify what we are good at and enjoy doing, and keep nurturing that talent instead of worrying and bothering about what we are not good at. If we are good at singing, we must focus on strengthening our singing capabilities instead of worrying about why we can't dance? If our natural instinct is singing, we can achieve the peak in signing effortlessly than by focusing on dancing.

How to activate the potential?

Activating your potential for greatness is a choice. Imagine that you are holding an acorn -if you leave this acorn and do not activate it by planting it in fertile soil and giving it sunlight and water and everything that it needs, that acorn would not be activated and would not become the great oak tree.

In the same way, you, your greatness must first be activated. And there are 8 steps to begin activating your potential for greatness should you want to live a life of meaning and fulfillment.

1) *Identify your passion:*

Put your ear down to your heart and listen hard. What are you passionate about? What you love the most? What you love doing with excitement even if you are not getting paid to do it? Who do you want to fight for? What books can you not stop reading? What moves you to tears? What stirs your soul? Your passions are not random; they are the ones that are your calling.

Think about what you want to be known for? Something will give you money, something will give you comfort. But that's not the point. What you choose to do will it give you a life? Living a life is not the problem, it is important if you consider your life is precious, you must make sure you make a wonderful life out of it. Spend some time with yourself and identify your gift, your talent that you can activate.

Ask people around you and the experts in that field to give honest feedback on your talent. For example, if you are passionate about singing, get feedback from people on your singing talent. Do they feel you are a good singer? Do the experts feel you have the talent that you are passionate about?

Finding your true passion is not very easy and it may take some time. Don't be restless.

2) *Align everything that you do in your life with your passions:*

Once you find your passion, align your actions with your passion to activate your greatness. When you do what you love, you give your best and maximize your potential.

3) Maximize the gifts that were given to you.

Everyone has some or the other talent and unique capabilities that we call a gift. I have gifts that perhaps you don't have, and you have gifts that perhaps I don't have. And that is on purpose. This is where I recommend you to be very selective about which parts of you are strengths and which are not. This is about strengthening your strengths and ignoring your weaknesses.

Ask yourself: what am I passionate about and uniquely gifted with. Those are your strengths; you ought to strengthen those. What would I happily stop doing because I'll never be great at it? Those are your weaknesses; ignore them.

4) Declare:

Set an intention and set that rocket of intention out into the universe. Create goal cards for everything that you want to achieve in your life. And read it in the morning and night to create new neural pathways of what you believe can be possible in the world. And believe it or not, these things do happen.

5) Believe:

Believe in the fact that you can create great things. Don't put a seed of doubt in your mind, you have done many great things in your life. What seemed impossible is now easy, from tying your shoes by yourself many years ago, to riding a bike, to all of the different things that you have done.

You have done some amazing things in your life, and you must begin to write them down. You will realize that earlier whenever you were presented with an opportunity to do something big, most of the time you said, "Oh, I don't have what it takes. I'm not good enough." But still, sometimes you were able to achieve it eventually.

So, instead start Saying, "It's easy", "I have all the qualities that are required to become a successful person." Protect yourself from people who are naysayers, don't listen to them and move on.

On your way to greatness; multiple forces will make you believe that you are not great and you are not special but at the same time there are signs and occurrences that will tell you otherwise choose wisely, believe in your gift, believe in your greatness and stay committed.

6) Commit to your dream, commit to your greatness:

Don't hesitate, commit to your greatness and take the first bold step. Once you are committed, you will find countless ideas and plans on your way.

7) Be brave:

Do the thing that you don't think you can do. This activates your maximum potential because magic does not happen within your comfort zone. If you could have achieved greatness within your current comfort zone, you would have already.

This is about stepping out of the familiar; this is about being slightly uncomfortable and daring to be courageous even though perhaps no one else is believing in you.

8) Expect:

Expect great things to happen, expect great results even when what you want is not showing up. I have a mantra that I would like you too to adopt. The mantra is, on a daily basis, "I am positively expecting great results no matter what I see in front of me. I know that the Universe is rearranging itself for my best interest right now." You say this all the time, and by saying this, you are allowing yourself to be in this place of positive expectation that changes your personal vibration and allows good things to come into your life.

Unleashing the true potential; The Hedgehog concept:

"There are two types of people in this world: hedgehogs and foxes." wrote Isaiah Berlin in his famous essay.

"The fox knows many things, but the hedgehog knows one big thing."

The fox is cunning, smart, very fast, sneaky and always in search of new strategies to beat the hedgehog and win his share of the forest.

The hedgehog, on the other hand, knows one big thing and uses only one strategy but executes it to perfection. Whatever the fox tries, the hedgehog defends himself with what he knows how to do best.

So, when they face each other, the fox tries a new strategy, but the hedgehog always wins. No matter what the fox tries, the hedgehog just curls up into a ball, exposes his spikes, and finally, the fox gives up.

In real life, foxes are those who always try new strategies to achieve their goals. Hedgehogs, on the other hand, are those who stick to a simple strategy and process. Hedgehogs are consistent. They trust the process, and they methodically work towards achieving their "dream job."

How do you become Hedgehog?

Every great company and great people within them follows the 'Hedgehog strategy' to go from mediocrity to greatness.

The Hedgehog concept is shared by Jim Colin in his book 'Good to Great'. A simple concept that requires deep understanding of the intersection of circles that talk about the following:

1) What are you deeply passionate about? (Passion)
2) What you can be the best in the world at, and (Talent)
3) What best drive your resources or economic engine? (Value)

Discovering the intersection is your 'hedgehog' or unleashing the true potential. Finding your hedgehog is not easy and may take some time as it has to be tried and tested in various situations and scenarios.

If you focus on just 'Passion' and 'Talent' then you will not create what is truly valuable to the society.

If you focus on 'Talent' and 'Value' then you will not be able to tap into your 'passion' which is a great motivator to push you out of your comfort zone and achieve greatness.

If you focus on 'Passion' and 'Value' and completely ignore

the 'Talent' then you will not be able to reach your true potential.

In order to tap to your true potential and achieve greatness, you must discover all 3 circles.

Did you find your hedgehog?

Exercise:

1) What are you truly passionate about?
2) What you want to be remembered for?
3) Are you committed to your passion?

Chapter 3

THE EASIEST AND MOST DIFFICULT WAY TO PERSONAL TRANFORMATION

"Quality of thoughts determines the quality of your life."

Do you know the difference between people who are successful and ones who are not? Do you know why it's easier for someone to achieve the heights of success whereas others are working hard to get that, yet they have not been able to reach where they want to?

Fundamentally, the most critical component of the process is thought. What differentiates a human with other species is the power of thinking. We have the power to create and destroy based on our thoughts. Our thoughts are very powerful and responsible for everything that happens in our life. Our thoughts create our destiny. The power of our thoughts is so immense that we can use the same power to create happiness and success, or sickness and failures. And the choice for what we want to create remains on us.

To understand how to create thoughts and how to take measurable steps towards our thoughts to perform at our best, we will take a little help from the 'Law of Attraction'.

You can have what you want:

It's very important here to understand the Law of Attraction, it is the most important law and works for everyone, everywhere and every time. It responds to your thoughts and simply gives you what you are thinking about. If you can think of performing with your peak-potential you will end up identifying your true potential and will surely be performing at the peak.

Our life, so far, is a reflection of our past thoughts. We attract what we think about so all the great things achieved so far are the result of our good thoughts in the past and what's not great in life so far is also the result of our thoughts that were not great. Now, you may think that you have never thought of this but your predominant thoughts have brought you where you currently are in your life. So we have to be very careful with our thoughts as we attract what we think about.

Law of attraction also says, Like attracts like, once you create the thought of performing at peak, you will start attracting the likes.

Magnetic effect of Thoughts:

Our thoughts have a frequency and magnetic effect. When we think about something, these thoughts are sent out into the Universe, and they magnetically attract like things that are on the same frequency. The law of attraction works every time, everywhere and with every person.

Isn't it amazing? Just think about what you want and the Universe will attract it to your life. Think about your dream house, dream car, dream career and what not and you will get that. Now the question is why everybody is not living the life of their dream? And why they don't have what they want. Everyone wants to see themselves successful rather than being a mediocre.

Why People don't get what they want?

The reason people do not have what they want is because they focus more on what they 'don't want' instead of 'what they want' Our subconscious mind, which is 90% powerful, doesn't understand any difference between imagination and reality so we have to be very careful with our thoughts and start imagining

'What we want' instead of 'what we don't want'. The Universe only focuses on your thoughts, not on your negative words like 'No', 'Don't', 'Not', etc.

Say "I want to be on time" instead of saying "I don't want to be late".

Say, "I want to succeed" Instead of saying "I don't want to fail".

Law is absolutely clear and it responds to your thoughts, it doesn't understand what's good or bad. It only responds to the signal that you are emitting into the universe. It is receiving your thoughts and reflecting back the same thoughts to your life.

All thoughts emerge in our mind and nobody is permitted to host any thought in our mind without our permission. We have to act like a guardian of our mind and take the responsibility to choose our thoughts.

Now the question is can we control or master our thoughts? How our thoughts help us in Identifying our true potential? Is it possible to perform at the peak with the power of thoughts?

The answer to all these questions is 'yes'. We can certainly change our life by changing our thoughts. By changing our thoughts, we can change our life and amplify our performance in any area of our life.

Having a mind full of positive thoughts is essential for any individual to unleash their true potential and perform at the peak level. An individual with a positive mental attitude can contribute significantly towards various areas of life whereas it's vice versa for somebody with a negative mental attitude.

Thoughts create our thinking style:

The type of thoughts (positive or negative) that we create determine our thinking style and eventually, our life surrounds the way we think. Our thinking guides us on how we are doing in our life. There are different thinking styles that individuals are operating in and it has a significant impact on how they are performing in various areas of their life. Here are the characteristics of 4 different thinking styles:

1) **Defeatist thinking style:** Individuals with 'Defeatist' thinking styles are dominated by negative and unproductive communication with self. They are surrounded by worry, frustration and fear most of the time. This thinking pattern allows them to continue dwelling with negativity.

2) **Sustainer Thinking Style:** Individuals with 'Sustainer' thinking style love to maintain the status quo and ignore the new idea or give reasons that it will never work, or will be shot down by Managers/Directors or by others. Instead of focusing on challenging the status quo with new and innovative ideas, they love to be in status-quo and it kills their creativity.

3) **Dreamer thinking style:** Individuals with this thinking style keep generating new ideas every now and then. It's not that they put a lot of effort generating those ideas, rather these ideas keep coming effortlessly. Most of these thoughts let them think about enormous possibilities out of nowhere and this keeps them very excited. If you have these sorts of thoughts keep coming to your mind then you are likely to stay

ahead in the race of your professional careers and continue to evolve. These sorts of thoughts help you in identifying your potential which in the case of the first 2 thinking styles wasn't possible.

4) **Opportunistic thinking style:** Ideas are worthless unless they are being acted upon. Once individuals are in the dreamer-thinking mode alloyed with massive action, they are on the path of peak performance. Under this thinking style, individuals are not just allowing ideas to emerge rather they put those ideas into action to transform their dreams into reality. People with this thinking style see positives, they are willing to do everything until they succeed, enthusiastic and positive about ideas and execution. They have an extremely positive attitude with a can-do approach.

What is your thinking style?

What is your thinking style and how it impacts your performance? Your effort is to eventually shift your thinking style to 'opportunists' because this is where the growth lies, this is where you identify your potential and your peak performance emerges.

Change thinking style

Now we realize that how a change in thinking style can change the outcome that we want to achieve in our life. Here are the steps to follow to change your thinking style:

1) **Be aware of your thinking style:** Ask yourself, which thinking style you have been operating from so far and how it has impacted the result. You will certainly find your thinking

style that emerges with your thoughts is the core reason for what you are today.

2) **Revisit where you want to be:** Revisit your goal and evaluate whether the current thinking style can take you there or not? You have to act like a guard on which 'thought' to allow to enter in our mind and which thought you have to restrict. If your goal is to move to performance enhancement mode in various areas of your life then you have to accept and take action to move from defeatist/sustainer to dreamer/ opportunists thinking style.

3) **Switch to Dreamer and eventually opportunistic thinking style:** Keep exploring various possibilities and generate new ideas. Don't just be in the status quo, try to come up with innovative ideas that can take you where you really wish to go. Once you have those ideas, put them into action and you will see the enormous potential that you have.

While it's easier to be in defeatist/sustainer thinking style but being aware of this itself is powerful and mandatory to have us shift to dreamer/opportunities thinking style eventually. Opportunistic thinking style is what we all want to be in and that's where we are able to perform with our potential.

Take charge of your Thoughts:

Be the master of your mind, and take charge. Keep your mind calm by practicing meditation and strengthen your mind with powerful thoughts. Be an active guard of your thoughts and whenever any negative thought comes across just say 'Not allowed' and convert them into positive and let them enter. If you want positive things to happen, focus on positive thoughts. Psychologists are convinced that our life moves in the direction of our most dominant thoughts.

"Your life today is a result of your thinking yesterday. Your life tomorrow will be determined by what you think today."

– John C Maxwell.

Chapter 4

THIS IS WHAT HOLDS YOU BACK...DITCH THEM AND UNLEASH YOUR POTENTIAL

"Whatever you believe is true is true even if it is not true."

- Saji Ijiyemi

Do you feel the sense of unworthiness, helplessness or hopelessness? Have you ever felt irrational doubts or fear? Do you feel something is holding you back from taking any decision that could have taken your personal and professional life at an entirely different level? Do you have the mental blocks like "I'm not good enough" "I don't deserve it" "I can't do this"?

2 weightlifters of the same category have the same weight to lift. They have identical training routines, same coach and similar physical capabilities. One of them believes he can lift the weight and the other one believes he can't. Which one is more likely to be successful? 2 engineers graduated from the same college, taught by the same teachers with a similar level of mental capabilities. One of them believes he can code very well, whereas, the other one feels he can't. Which one is more likely to code well? There is a link between mind and body, what you think and BELIEVE will affect how you behave and perform.

You might not be aware of the reason for these feelings but the simple reason for you to have all these feelings is because your mind is coded and programmed that way. Each one of us has a tremendous amount of potential and we deserve to live a wonderful life but the way we are programmed or coded is the real blockage that is holding us back. Empowering beliefs help us unleash our true potential and push us to perform at our peak.

Belief of the 4-Minute-Mile Barrier:

Before 6th May 1954, no one in history had run one mile in less than 4 minutes. None of them believed that this was even physically possible. A lot of experts also believed that it was beyond the capability of any human body to run a mile in less than 4 minutes. For several years this belief was perceived as a fact, a lot of athletes tried to break this barrier but none of them got success.

On May 6th 1954, an athlete, powered with belief, named Rodger Bannister, ran one mile in 3 minutes and 59 seconds. By doing so, he not just created a world record but also broke a false belief that stayed alive in the minds of thousands of runners for several years. Bannister was powered with this belief and his body responded with this belief to make it happen.

A year later, many other runners also broke this barrier and it's no more a belief now. It clearly says that a barrier was never ever there, it just existed in the mind and the mind was programmed in a way to make this belief as fact.

What is a belief?

A belief is something that we consider to be a fact whether it is actually true or not. We are, for the most part of our life, controlled by these beliefs that run our life. Belief is what and how we have programmed our subconscious mind. Most of the decisions and actions we are taking in our life are based on how we are coded or programmed.

Beliefs play an important role to run our life, it gives us the necessary strength in reaching our goals. Beliefs dictate what we consider to be possible or not.

For example, let's say you were raised in a middle-class family and constantly struggled financially during your life. Every time you asked money from your family, you heard, "Money doesn't grow on trees". Therefore, your subconscious learnt this and might have developed a belief such as "making money is very difficult" and/or "You have to work very hard to make money".

How beliefs are formed?

Beliefs are generally formed based on our experiences and what people (especially our parents, teachers, elders and people around us) told us to be true. During our day-to-day life, we also observe several things around us (like what people are saying, how they are behaving and/or what point of view that they have for any particular matter) that helps us form our beliefs. We were completely a clean slate when we entered this world as a baby. Our parents and environment played a major role in making us believe in almost everything that is stored in our subconscious mind as beliefs. These beliefs are installed in our mind like a computer program and once the program is installed, our mind works based on that programming.

Here's the small story of how beliefs are formed. When we were a kid, we saw a cockroach approaching us and we kept getting excited, assuming it's a sort of toy coming to us. But as soon as our mom saw that cockroach approaching closer to us... she hit the cockroach saying this is bad, hence, we learnt that cockroaches are bad and can be dangerous. That's how we form various beliefs when were a child.

As we continued to grow, we met new friends and teachers, eventually, our beliefs continued to get influenced. For example, our teachers told us that "we are not good enough" and if the same is repeated over and again we start believing this as a fact.

As you enter adulthood and if some of your friends tell you that "you are not cool" then you get programmed that way and because your subconscious keeps hearing this from your peers on regular basis without using any filters, it starts believing the same even if you are one of the coolest guys.

When we accept something as a fact, it gets stored in our subconscious mind and it triggers the action based on our belief because our subconscious mind doesn't know whether this belief is true or not.

If somehow, we can transport empowering beliefs in our subconscious and remove negative belief patterns then we can certainly make positive changes in our life.

Belief confirmation:

Once the belief is formed, our subconscious mind starts gathering the evidence to validate this belief to be true. In the process, we completely ignore all the data that is opposite to our belief.

For example; if you have a belief that "your friend is not capable", you will find all the evidence to validate this belief. You will only be looking for his incapability and won't even focus on what he is capable of. You won't make any conscious effort to do this, your subconscious mind will continue to do this automatically based on your belief. It will only look for information that it has deep-rooted beliefs and will continue to ignore the information that is contradictory to the beliefs.

How beliefs affect our behavior:

Beliefs shape our world and have a significant impact on our life. Once the beliefs are installed, we can see the world through those beliefs. Your positive beliefs about the same world can make this whole world beautiful, wonderful, happy and abundant whereas your negative belief can make the whole world ugly, fearful and dangerous for you. Remember, the world around you is the same but what makes the difference is your belief system. If your beliefs about any particular thing are positive, your subconscious mind will trigger you to take the action in your life that can help you flourish in that particular area. Whereas, it is vice versa if our beliefs about that particular area are negative. Your positive beliefs help you unleash your true potential and perform according to that.

Let's say, you once failed in learning something in your childhood and your teacher and people around you remarked that "you are not a good learner". While for your teacher this was just feedback and a normal statement but you have started believing it's true. Now you enter your professional career with the same deep-rooted belief and there is a situation where you are required to learn a new technology. You do try to learn but you fail on the first attempt. You consult a few friends and they encourage you to try once more, though you don't want to because you believe that you are not a good learner. But with their persuasion, you decide to give it another go and with the same deep-rooted belief that "you are not a good learner" and guess, what would happen? In your next attempt, you would experience yet another failure. However, on the other hand, one of your colleagues, with the belief that "everything is possible" is able to learn this with half of the efforts that you put into it.

Think about the impact of these 2 different beliefs that can influence your professional career and growth going forward. The ones with a 'not' severely impact your performance and hold you back in identifying your true potential. Following are some of the examples of Negative beliefs

"You are not good enough."

"You can't do this."

"This is too hard."

"Being excellence is not my cup of tea."

At the same time, positive beliefs give you the power to stay positive, help you to keep unleashing your potential and perform at your peak. Following are some of the examples of positive beliefs

"Everything is Possible."

"I can learn to succeed."

"I always produce results."

"If someone has done it, I can do that too."

By holding limiting beliefs, we limit our performance and growth in our professional career and life. If we are holding a senior position in any of the organization then our self-limiting beliefs impact not just our performance but also the performance of our team and the entire organization. When we have self-limiting beliefs as an executive, we can't inculcate the team with empowering beliefs. Hence it's a recipe for limiting the growth.

Are our limiting beliefs helpful? No, Right? Then change it! And, yes, you can change your limiting beliefs!

How to reprogram our mind for Limiting beliefs:

You can reprogram your deep-rooted limiting beliefs that are holding you back from pursuing and achieving our dreams and goals. Remember, your beliefs are what you believe to be true, not necessarily they are true. So you can certainly change them.

If you have empowering and positive beliefs that continue to fuel you with required energy and motivation, no need to change... Hip, Hip, and Hurrah! You are all set, continue to strengthen them and keep growing.

But if your beliefs are limiting ones and holding you back, you must change them without waiting as it keeps you in low energy, holds you back and hampers the quality of action that you are expected to take for your dreams and goals. Here's a 6-step process to reprogram your mind:

1) **Be aware about your belief:** Look at the key areas of your life i.e. health, wealth, career, and relationship and identify which area of your life is not meeting the goals that you have set for those areas. Which area of your life you are not happy with? Which area of your life do you feel is incompetent and powerless?

These are some tough questions, so be honest and deep-dive to get an answer to those, it may take some time but you will certainly get those.

For example; if you feel you are not doing as good in your career as you want to, identify the limiting beliefs that you have for your career. Ask these questions to get the answer. What has stopped you so far in your career? What is something that is standing between you and success? Why are you not been able to grow?

Keep observing the thoughts that are stopping you to take action. Once you identify and acknowledge your limiting beliefs find out how those beliefs are formed, find out how this has impacted you so far and why are you believing in those beliefs.

For example; if your limiting belief is "I'm not good enough" then think about how this belief was formed. This deep-rooted belief that you will never be good enough comes from your programming and experience. Your subconscious mind remembered this experience and made you believe that you are not good enough.

Ask yourself, how this belief has impacted you and why you have this belief. Are you believing in this because someone told you over and again? And that someone is somebody who you feel has more knowledge than you?

2) **Question your belief and turnaround:** Start questioning your limiting belief and you will begin to doubt your beliefs. You may ask these questions and keep doubting your belief:

   a. What makes me feel that I'm not good enough?

   b. Have I never been good enough in my career so far?

   c. What makes me believe this?

   d. How can someone judge me with 100% accuracy?

   e. Why am I believing in something that somebody told me?

All these questions will create doubt and you will start feeling that maybe this is my wrong belief that I'm not good enough.

3) **Associate massive pain with not changing your existing limiting belief:** After raising the question you have already started doubting your belief and now you can associate the massive pain of how these limiting beliefs can impact you in the future if you don't change. For change to happen, you need motivation and pain can be one of the greatest motivations to change your limiting beliefs. Here's how you can associate pain to your limiting beliefs:

My career will be negatively impacted if I continue with this belief,

How I will be able to take care of my family,

How my social image is impacted if I won't grow,

How I will fulfill the dreams of mine and my children.

Once you associate enough pain to our limiting belief, your subconscious mind is tempted to change your beliefs and time comes when you say… enough is enough! I can't continue with this belief anymore and that is the time for immediate massive change. This is how our mind works which we have to understand and act accordingly. Even if you feel the change is fearful, feel the fear and do it anyway.

4) **Reframe and reinforce:** After you take a call to change your limiting belief to empowering one, reframe your limiting belief "you are not good enough" to something like "I'm capable to do anything". Similarly, you can reframe your other limiting beliefs to empowering ones. Just by reframing

you will get enough energy to go ahead with them and live your life of dreams.

5) **Conditioning:** Once you reframe your belief, Conditioning of empowering belief is the key to make sure the change you create is consistent and lasts long. Code your subconscious mind with new empowering belief. Train your subconscious mind on the pleasure that this new belief is going to give it to you once it forms part of your belief system. Keep reminding your subconscious mind over and again for various positives until the neural pathway is created for the new empowering belief.

Also, continue to believe in your empowering belief and imagine doing it over and again until you see this empowering belief is helping you to come out of pain and enjoy the pleasure. You may not get the result immediately as it takes some time to neglect the effect of your deep-rooted beliefs that are a part of your system for a long time. But if you continue with your new empowering belief over and again with emotional intensity, your mind will experience the new way of achieving the result.

For example; when you go to the gym to build your muscle, you can't just go for a few days and get the result. You make your mind aware of the benefits of the results for being consistent and that benefit makes you follow the workout on a regular basis. Without conditioning your subconscious mind, your mind can't make this belief as part of your system.

6) **Mastermind:** Continue to be in the group of like-minded people or community that encourages you to continue with empowering beliefs. Having surrounded by like-minded

people is always helpful and adds fuels to the body and mind for success.

Having negative coding in your mind is extremely harmful and it severely impacts the growth in various areas of your life without making you realize why it's happening. Once you change those beliefs to empowering ones, you can't even imagine the transformation that you are going to experience and enjoy.

Therefore, it's time for you to Act Now. Ask yourself, what are your limiting beliefs. Identify your various limiting beliefs that are holding you back and empower yourself with empowering beliefs!

Must have empowering Beliefs:

1) I have all the qualities that are required to be a successful person.
2) I have everything within me.
3) Everything is possible.
4) I am born to Succeed.
5) Everything happens for a reason.
6) There is no failure it's feedback only.
7) I can find a way.
8) I always produce results.
9) The Universe is always helping me.
10) Being successful is easy.
11) I am born to be a genius.

Exercise to install empowering belief:

1) Identify your self-limiting beliefs.
2) How your self-limiting beliefs have impacted your life?
3) How your life will be after 5 years if you don't change your self-limiting beliefs?
4) How your life will be after 5 years if you replace your self-limiting beliefs with empowering beliefs and condition your mind for those?

Chapter 5

THE GAME-CHANGER... MINDSET OR HEARTSET?

"Eliminate the mindset of CAN'T! Because you CAN do it!"

- Tony Horton

Michael Jordan is one of the most famous basketball players in the world, though, he wasn't always a star. He didn't make it to his high school basketball team because he was too short and wasn't good enough. He could have quit, but he didn't, why?

If you have ever had some goals and dreams that didn't come true, you are not alone. More than 90% of people never achieve what they set for. But yes, about 10% do achieve their goals. Why? What sets apart those who accomplish great things from those who are only dreaming of accomplishing? Why few people always try new things and push themselves into uncharted territory whereas others are stuck with what they know? Why do few people believe that anyone can be anything whereas others believe they are not made for it?

The answer to all these 'Whys' lies in Mindset. Yes, it's not intelligence, creativity or appetite for risk that sets apart one set of people from the next, instead, it's the mindset that makes them accomplish great things, perform the best they want to and do wonders.

Now the question is what mindset is, and how to determine what type of mindset these 2 sets of people have? Mindset is nothing but a set of assumptions and beliefs, it is the way our brain functions or the way we set our mind to deal with different situations.

Michael Jordan had the mindset to continue and get better. He was out practicing each day before most people were even out of bed. And because of this, he not only made the team the following year, but he went on to become the greatest player of all time and a true champion. The question that comes to our minds is:

Can we all learn to have the mindset of a champion and perform in our day-to-day life the way he did in the basketball court?

Having the right mindset is very important. It can help you perform better, grow in your life and accomplish what you want and reach where you want to be. Whereas, not having the right mindset can make you feel stuck and not grow with the pace you want to.

Growth Mindset Vs Fixed Mindset:

Carol Dweck, psychologist Stanford University has got a lot deeper on the subject and her major contribution is the distinction between fixed mindset and growth mindset. There are 2 types of people in terms of mindset:

One of the biggest attributes of someone with a growth mindset is that they believe their basic intelligence and abilities can be changed with consistent efforts. They are not afraid of challenges and continue to increase their efforts when things come harder.

Say a software engineer with a growth mindset is not good at team management instead of saying "I'm not good at it". Now, since this engineer has a growth mindset, he would simply say "I will learn how to manage team" because he knows that the amount of effort he puts into something is directly related to how much success he is going to get out of it. Individuals with a growth mindset believe talent comes through effort. They believe anyone can be good at anything; that their abilities can be developed through dedication, perseverance, and the right strategy.

In a **fixed mindset**, individuals believe they are either born with talent or they are not. They are either naturally good at something, or they are not. They can't learn and they are afraid of challenges. They view intelligence as a fixed trait and feel criticized when given feedback. They believe inborn talent determines success.

Here are some interesting day-to-day situations that tell us about which mindset we are carrying in some of the day-to-day work situations:

1) Feedback by Manager:

How do you feel when you get feedback from your manager on the recent project you delivered that it didn't meet with the quality standards and your manager feels you have not done a great job on it?

Is your response like you are not talented enough for the job, this is the best you can do, you can't learn this doing better than what you have done, other colleagues of the team are not supportive, spend rest of the day cribbing and complaining and you will even start looking for another job? If your response matches with any of these then you are trapped into a fixed mindset.

The growth mindset's response is to do a self-evaluation of your performance, get constructive feedback, identify the areas that need improvement, and figure out the strategy to get better, work on this, apply these to your day-to-day work and be a better performer.

2) New project or task:

What's your take when you have been given the responsibility of new and challenging project that requires new technology to implement that you haven't learnt so far? Do you think "I'm not capable to do it" "I can't learn the technology that this project requires"?

OR Do you think, "Wow, what a wonderful opportunity to learn this new technology" "How can I learn this faster to have quality deliverable within the timeline"?

The former approach is a fixed mindset whereas later one is a growth mindset.

3) Praising subordinates:

Everyone loves praises, especially when they perform exceptionally well. Praises are the real fuel and motivation to continue to do what they are doing. How do you praise your subordinates? Are you following the growth mindset route or the fixed mindset route?

If you acknowledge their effort by saying "You are so smart" "You are intelligent", it will give them the label or identity of them being 'Smart' and 'intelligent' which is a fixed mindset.

Growth mindset praises are very effective as they don't give them any identity, label or talent rather it praises their effort, strategy or process. So instead of saying "You are smart" growth mindset could say "The process that you have followed and the strategy that you have implemented is quite incredible. Your extensive efforts on the project are also a reason for the project being delivered with such a high quality. Very well done!"

While we have seen in various situations that the individuals, teams and organizations with a growth mindset have performed much better, grown way better and sustained over the long term than the ones with a fixed mindset.

Studies and researches have proven over and again that the brain is not a fixed entity and it can be developed with continuous efforts and proper strategies. Though, no study says that it can be developed at the same rate for 2 different individuals or everyone can be the best in any specific skills but it's quite sure that with continuous efforts, people can get better in any skill.

Learning and practicing are the key:

Learning and practicing are an important element to continue to perform better. How do you think the 'God of Cricket', Sachin Tendulkar achieved his success over a long period of time, is it just his God-gifted natural talent? No, it's not just that, there is something else too, natural talent can make you perform on a few occasions but to sustain over a long period of time, you need something else too. Sachin continued to learn new tricks and practice harder for every single match and for every single inning, he continued to read the strategy of every single bowler and every single team. He knew challenges are a part of any professional career and he had set his mindset in a way that made him one of the best performers for a very long period of time.

Almost everyone believes that having the growth mindset increases the probability of identifying your peak potential and growing your professional career way better in the long run than in the fixed mindset. With several advantages and importance of having the growth mindset, those want to grow in their careers and perform better are eager to learn how to have their mindset shift from fixed to growth.

Before we share the secret on how to make this happen, it's important to understand that developing a growth mindset is easy, but easy things are difficult, there are challenges and it requires efforts, however, it's achievable over time. Remember, the brain is adaptable to improve through continuous learning and new information. Our brain can function much better when we are working out of our comfort zone during challenging situations.

Why it's recommended to have a growth mindset:

"Once your mindset changes, everything on the outside will change along with it."

- Steve Maraboli.

With innovation and automation being the priority for most of the industries, Robots taking over basic manual operations, automation has substantially taken over various functions where manual efforts were involved. Therefore, it's important to continue to develop and learn in newer areas for future-ready jobs. With all these innovations, challenges and situations are going to be entirely different than what we have had over the last few decades or so. Hence, it's important to keep ourselves in the growth-minded zone and be ready to develop new skills, change behavior, improve performance and accept challenges.

How to develop growth Mindset:

Now the question is how to develop the growth mindset to continue to evolve and perform at our peak in our professional careers? Changing your mindset doesn't happen by accident. It happens by choice, and these 7 steps should help get you on the right track:

1) **Self-talk:** Talk to yourself and if you feel you have the fixed mindset voice, think on how it's impacting the progress in our life. Also, think of how much progress is possible if the choice is given to have them convert into a growth mindset.

2) **Check your belief system:** Check your belief system if you feel it's not working, change it. (Already discussed this in relevant chapter-2)

3) **Choice of voice:** After you realize you have a fixed mindset voice, immediately realize that you have the choice and voice back with a growth mindset.

4) **Ask for Feedback:** Praise is highly motivational and can motivate everyone to high-performing individuals when given correctly. If we want to shift from fixed to growth mindset, we should get constructive feedback, accept the negative feedback, take it positively as a tool to improve upon the areas that are necessary are the keys to grow further in our careers and day-to-day life.

5) **Growth Mindset Action:**

   a. *Learn & Apply:* Identify the areas that help you grow and constantly focus on learning those. Applying those learning to practice is the key.

   b. *Constantly push yourself to Stretch Zone:* Being in the growth mindset requires extra efforts and we have to come out of our comfort zone to learn new things. And yes, consistency is the key. There will certainly be some challenges initially in terms of schedule and efforts but if you overcome those for some time it will continue to help you for the rest of your life.

c. *Learning Vs Performance Goal:* While this may not sound so bad, the problem is that people with a fixed mindset are more likely to create a performance approach or performance-avoidance goals. Setting learning goals helps you in taking new challenges, experimenting, effort and, ultimately, improvement. It's time to place a stronger emphasis on goals that will ensure you are always striving to learn, improve and try new things.

d. *Modeling:* Look for the best people in the area that you want to learn and adopt their thinking patterns and mindset. It's not just copying as it is but adopting what works for you. For example, if you want to be a successful business leader, you can role modeled successful business leaders to a certain degree.

6) Magic of the 3-letter word 'Yet'

Power of words like 'Yet' or 'Not yet' is really magical and can boost motivation.

Always put 'Yet' at the end of your sentence. When we believe we can't do something "yet", we implant the idea that it is possible. We only need to keep trying.

"I can't do it"

"I can't do it…Yet"

"I'm not good enough"

"I'm not good enough…Yet"

The magical word 'Yet' makes you feel that you need to put a little bit more effort into this instead of feeling that you are nothing and going nowhere. By using 'Yet' you understand that you are on a learning curve and with some more efforts, changed strategies and process you can get better.

7) **Protect growth Mindset:** Protect your growth mindset and make sure anybody with a fixed mindset doesn't let you down by saying you are not good enough. Remember, you can be anyone or anything you want to be as long as you set up your mindset to it.

Story:

One of the renowned technology companies 'X' was struggling to get quality projects despite their efforts. On a bright sunny day one of the clients 'Y Inc.', from United States of America approached them to work on the first phase of the project that required the latest technology such as Artificial intelligence, Machine Learning, Drone technology, blah blah… After the kick-off meeting with client, Mr. Michael, CTO of the company 'X', invited 2 of their 'Tech Leads', Sam and Mac (along with their Project Managers) to discuss on the project and to get an understanding on which one of them was confident to take the ownership of quality deliverables of the project within the timeline.

Mr. Sam, after understanding the detailed scope of the project responded as follows;

"I've never worked on a project with such complex technology and I don't have skills to work on this" and "I don't think I will be able to learn those skills with ease."

"There are too many challenges in this project with a tight deadline that requires me to stretch my schedule on a regular basis which is quite uncomfortable."

After having this discussion with Sam, Michael invited Mac to get his inputs;

"I've never worked on a project with such complexity but this is a wonderful opportunity for me to get the experience of working on such a latest technology."

"I don't have the depth of experience on these technologies but I will put all my efforts to learn them as learning these are not very difficult."

"I love challenging projects and if needed, I will stretch my schedule to meet with all the quality and timeline that this project can require."

What happened next?

Sam continued to work on the same technologies for other small projects within his comfort zone. He was enjoying his routine work without much discomfort to his schedule.

Whereas Mac was passionate about learning all the new technologies that the project required, he kept learning and applying those on this project. While doing so, he didn't even realize that for several weeks he worked way beyond his schedule. He kept getting feedback from his CTO and other senior colleagues and continued to alter his strategies based on the feedback to deliver the best he could. There were several challenges and a few failures in between but he used all of them to learn and move on.

Outcome:

With his consistent efforts and the right strategy, Mac was able to deliver the quality deliverables within the timeline. The client was very happy and based on the output of the project, 'Y Inc.' signed a $5M contract with 'X' company for the next 3 years that shaped the future of the company.

The company was very happy with the performance of Mr. Sam and awarded a bonus of $50,000/- and promoted him to Director, Technology.

Analysis:

Mr. Sam had a fixed mindset and his growth was severely impacted because of this. Neither he was able to find his true potential nor was he able to perform at peak. His meager growth was no surprise for anybody.

Mr. Mac, with his growth mindset, was able to identify his true potential, he learnt new skills and was able to perform at his peak when challenges knocked on his door. It's not that he didn't have a tough time in between but he took them as good learning opportunities and continued to move on.

No doubt about it, as the name suggests; the growth mindset gives you growth and the fixed mindset keeps you stuck where you are.

Do you want to identify your true potential and perform at your peak? You know which mindset can have you have this!

The decision is yours!

If the mindset is so important, what about the heartset?

"A good head and good heart are always a formidable combination."

- Nelson Mandela

In our previous story, is it just the mindset of Mac that made him successful? Most of the time, we emphasize a lot on our 'mindset'. We focus on the mindset of leaders to accomplish any goal, mindset of champions to perform at peak, mindset of winners to draw success in our life. While there is no denial that mindset does matter and plays a significant role in the overall success of individuals. But what about the heartset? Mindset is important to be successful but it will not give us everlasting happiness because happiness is determined by our heartset.

Mindset is just one side of the coin and heartset is the other side of the same coin. Simply stating, mindset is the way we think about the things that affect us and heartset is the way we feel about the things that affect us. Mindset determines our thought pattern and heartset determines our emotional pattern.

If you are being told to do the most exciting activity that you can possibly think of, how would you feel?

Now, if you are being told to do something that you don't love doing, something that you fear about and something that is outside of your comfort zone but doing that thing is mandatory to keep your life happier. How would you feel?

I am sure you would love doing what is most exciting and try your best to avoid the activity that you don't love doing. That's what the heartset is. It's your deep emotional attachment to person, place or thing. It's one of the most prominent inner drives to achieving a goal at all costs. Heartset is your heart's desire and it's a necessity like having oxygen to breathe.

Having a growth mindset helps accomplish much in a lifetime but it has a limitation especially when the going gets tougher. During a tough and challenging time, your inner drive and emotional connection make the difference and that's where the heartset comes into play. Heartset accepts no failure, no quit; it's unconditional passion despite all challenges.

Mac, in our story, not just completed his project with his growth mindset, his emotional connection and feeling of happiness after the project getting accomplished, staying courageous when going gets tough had also contributed significantly.

Having the right balance between the heartset and mindset is important if you want to have success accompanied by happiness.

Feeling of courage and enthusiasm when things are challenging and scary, feeling of abundance rather than scarcity, are some of the examples of a good heartset.

To sum it up, mindset is half the magic and it gets complete when it is accompanied by heartset.

Chapter 6

DO YOU KNOW WHY YOU BEHAVE-HOW YOU BEHAVE?

Do you remember any moment or situation on any day when you have messed up with the things that you have been doing quite comfortably with a lot of ease on any other day? It may be your business meeting, interview, sales presentation, examination or dealing with any of your family member. There may also be a day when you are completely in flow, everything is falling in just perfectly and it seems nothing can go wrong on that particular day.

What's the difference? You being the same person, with the similar level of intelligence, knowledge in similar situations but why these two behaviors are different? Why are you an absolute disaster on one day and extremely remarkable on other days?

Story-1

Sam, One of the best sales managers and topmost closure for his company, was almost ready to go to his sales meeting when he had an argument with his wife just before leaving. That made him completely upset and broke. As the meeting started Sam's physiology was extremely negative and he wasn't been able to deliver what he was expected to. Guess why did it happen?

Story-2

Michael, a good salesperson (not as good as Sam is), before leaving for his sales meeting he had a quick 2-minute call with his wife and they ended up with an exchange of love. That ferried Michael in a supreme mood. As the meeting went by, Michael was able to deliver the best he could and his presentation was appreciated by his clients that made him generate a very good order.

What's the difference? Sam, despite being a better salesperson, wasn't been able to perform as well as Michael. Why?

It's because of the state they are in. Now the question is what is state? And how it impacts the behavior? State is the emotion we experience at that particular moment. It is the neuro-physiological process at any given point. It's your way of being in any moment. It's a sum total of thoughts + emotions + Physical energy. In layman's language, you can call it a mood, a cricketer may call it a form.

State can be resourceful or un-resourceful. When we are in a resourceful state, we feel confident, happy, love and joyful whereas we feel fearful, depress, confuse, angry, upset and sad while we're in an un-resourceful state.

State is very powerful, our behavior is the result of the state we are in. When we are in a resourceful state, we do the best with all the available resources which results in the right action. This can produce wonderful results that make us feel quite positive and happy. In a resourceful state, our performance is at its best and we can produce successful results.

When we are in un-resourceful state, our behaviors are filled up with frustration and anger that can severely impact the action we are taking and can damage the result. Though it may make us feel embarrassed and regretful later but it's too late to realize as this behavior might have resulted in something that has already done the damage.

Successful people are able to be in a resourceful state on a consistent basis. Being in a resourceful state is one of the big differentiators for them being successful and others are not. It's not that they are not in a un-resourceful state ever. But most of the time, they keep themselves in a resourceful state that empowers them to take action with the available resources in the best possible way which can do wonders for them.

Now the question is which state you are mostly in? Have you ever realized?

Since we know our behavior is the result of our state than why not be in a resourceful state all the time? Why can't we have behaviors that can have the right type of action, that can produce a successful result and do wonders all the time? The question is, is it possible to be in a resourceful state all the time OR if we are in an un-resourceful state, can we change our state to resourceful state? In the next section, we will deep-dive into how the state is formed, if it all it can be changed and how.

This is how state is formed:

Let's just understand how we perceive any event; we perceive the world through five senses i.e. See (Visual learning), Hear (Auditory learning), Touch (Kinesthetic learning), Smell (Olfactory learning) and Taste (Gustatory learning). Since we are working on our inner-self so we will be focusing on the first 3 senses only.

We don't store the world as it is perceived through our senses; rather we delete, distort or generalize the event through our senses before we store it in our memory, and after the filtration process of actual event, we store the event in our mind as our inner representation.

This inner representation is called PIR (Personal Internal Representation). PIR and actual event may entirely differ and most importantly each person may have different PIR for the same event. For example, 5 people meet one famous celebrity at the airport, now each person can have different PIR of that celebrity. This Personal Internal Representation which is stored in our mind triggers a Physiology and thus a State gets achieved which is the sum total of both PIR and Physiology.

Why to change State?

We come through various states in our day-to-day life. State management is the key to become highly effective and productive. If we are in a resourceful state we shouldn't be bothered about changing our state but if we are in un-resourceful state then we must change the state to perform at our peak. Those who are not able to manage their state are not in a position to utilize their true potential and are not able to perform the best they actually can. The 2 states, resourceful and un-resourceful, create a different type of behavior that directly impacts the result, hence changing the state can directly help to change the quality of results.

When you are in a resourceful state, you are always making good decisions, producing good behavioral actions and you perform up to your potential. But when you are in an un-resourceful state, you create hell out of heaven and do things that you shouldn't.

So if we can be in a resourceful state, we can produce wonderful results through our behavior, but the question is, is it possible to change the state immediately to get transformed from being depressed to being excited, being underconfident to confident or positive to negative? Do we have the power to change the STATE? Are we equipped by ourselves to change the state? And the answer to all these questions is YES! But how?

The next sections are very helpful in guiding us on how to change the STATE and do wonders in our day-to-day life.

Change your state in less than 5 seconds and be at your Peak State;

We all enjoy being in a resourceful state; though we can't be in a resourceful state all the time for various unavoidable reasons. But sometimes, we feel ourselves being trapped in an un-resourceful state. Isn't it amazing if we know how to shift from un-resourceful to resourceful state?

Changing the state can happen in seconds! Yes, that's true, it doesn't even take minutes! It happens so fast that we never ever thought of. State-change is magical and it's very simple but sometimes we look for very complicated solutions to our problem and feel these simple solutions can't be helpful!

Here's how we can change the state:

Awareness about your State: Being aware of which state you are in and which state you want to be in is the key component of State change. After the state is being identified we can now change the state as follows:

1) ***Neutralize the un-resourceful triggers:*** Identify the triggers that take you in an un-resourceful state. It may be something that someone did or memory or past experience. Identify those triggers and have the courage to deal with those without having those impacting you.

2) ***Change Physiology:*** Since you are in an un-resourceful state, your physiology is also un-resourceful, use 'as if' rule to change your physiology (facial expression, balance of the

spine, shoulder, breathing pattern, inner talk or do anything that circulates different chemical in your body).

Change your physiology 'AS IF' you are confident, look up, broaden your shoulder, wear a smile on your face, and your mind will immediately access the PIR of confidence that's already there in the mind. Thence, as soon as you will get confident PIR, you will suddenly start feeling in resourceful state.

Let's say you are upset for any reason and sitting with a negative body language. Now, if you immediately get up and stand tall as if you are confident then your mind will read your body language and start finding the PIR of confident feeling. As soon as it accesses your PIR for confident feeling, you will certainly see yourself from negative to Positive.

3) Ask better questions: Asking resourceful and powerful questions is one of the easiest and quickest ways to have your mind approach to those positive PIRs.

   i. What can I learn from this?

   ii. What's the most positive part of this experience?

   iii. How can I perform better under this situation?

   iv. How can I use this problem as an opportunity?

4) Change your thoughts: If your thinking pattern is negative, you can't feel good and that can drag you in an un-resourceful state. Therefore, change your thoughts, and have empowering thoughts to access positivity. Once you access your positivity, your mind will search the PIR of positive person that's already there in the mind and as soon as you will get a positive PIR, you will suddenly start feeling in a resourceful state.

5) ***Change your internal representation:*** Any state is the result of PIR that we make about an object or circumstances. By using our senses, we can change the mental picture. For example, for any fear, instead of exaggerating or terrifying that it really is, consciously reduce the size and impact of that fear and you will be amazed to see your emotions getting shifted in a few seconds.

Few Tips

1) Don't share or discuss your sadness with others. When you are sad and share the reasons for your sadness with multiple people, you are making your negative PIRs stronger which ultimately is driving your negative behavior and impacting your productivity and performance adversely.
2) Don't listen to sad songs when you are already upset, sad and disheartened. Listen to positive songs and positive talks when you are in un-resourceful state. As soon as your mind will listen to those it will gradually start feeling better and start searching for resourceful PIR. And as soon as it gets that, your state will turn from un-resourceful to resourceful.

Chapter 7

IT'S ABOUT YOU!

"Accept no one's definition of your life; define yourself."

- Harvey Fierstein

Self-Concept:

Self-concept is nothing but your overall idea and perception of who you are. It is your comprehensive personal evaluation of how you see yourself, how you value yourself and think and feel about yourself. Self-concept, is formed based on your knowledge about yourself, is very important and determines your performance in various areas of your life because you will act in the outer world based on your self-concept in your inner world. Every change you want to make in the outer world first starts with a change in your inner world.

Self-concept is developed right from childhood and early adulthood, though it can be changed later but it requires a lot of effort in changing the perception once it's formed.

Parts of Self-Concept

According to Carl Rogers, American psychologist, Self-concept has 3 parts, self-ideal, self-image and self-esteem:

Ideal-Self

Self-ideal is how you wish you could be or how you would like to see yourself. Self-ideal is made up of all qualities and values that you admire most and would like to have those to be a perfect person. Your self-ideal determines your behavior and skills you would like to learn and adopt. If your ideal-self has high standards, virtues and greater ambitious then you strive to live up to your ideal-self.

Self-Image

"A strong, positive self-image is the best possible preparation for success."

- Joyce Brothers

Self-image is how you see yourself, it is how you look in your inner-mirror. Your inner-image can have attributes like physical characteristics (tall, short, brown-eyes, fair complexion...., etc.), social roles (Student, husband, Director of marketing, Grandfather..., etc.), and personality traits (Generous, self-motivated, enthusiastic..., etc.). Based on your inner-image of yourself, you go out and perform in the external world. If you have a self-image of yourself as one of the confident speakers, the same will be reflected when you go on stage and deliver your speech.

Self-image and reality may not align perfectly, few may have inflated self-image than what they are whereas others may just focus on the flaws and weaknesses that others don't see at all.

Visualizing yourself with a stronger self-image is one of the powerful techniques to send your subconscious mind a command, which your subconscious mind accepts as an order and aligns your consistent actions with the self-image that you have created for yourself. For example, let's say you don't have a strong self-image as a speaker but if you visualize yourself with a strong self-image as a speaker then your subconscious mind gets a command. It then uses this command to have you perform better as a speaker when you are delivering your speeches.

How much you value yourself depends on whether your self-ideal and self-image are in congruence or incongruent.

Self-Esteem:

This is one of the most important components of your personality and hence it's being covered in greater detail here. Let's understand this with one example before we discuss the impact of self-esteem and how we can have high self-esteem to magnify our performance in various areas of our life.

Rahul is a software engineer whose skills are quickly recognized by his reporting manager. Rahul's analytical and problem-solving approach has been appreciated by all his peers. He gets on with his team very well and helps them wherever needed.

After a year of association, his manager recommends him for promotion and he has been given additional responsibilities. He performs very well on the new role but instead of giving credit to himself for his efforts, he continues to feel it just happened.

A year later, a position of technical manager opens and his manager recommends him to apply for that position because he feels Rahul has the skills to do well for that position. Rahul is quite shocked by this suggestion, and he feels he is not good enough for the role. So he doesn't apply and that position has been given to another employee within the same company at a better pay.

Earlier also, he found a number of reasons for not accepting the praises given by his peers, telling himself that he doesn't deserve it and anybody could have done that as well.

Why Rahul is like that? Does he have low self-esteem? In the current corporate world, many people are like Rahul. They reflect low self-esteem and not able to recognize the praises received from their colleagues. They feel too low for themselves which is impacting their career progression and financial growth. They don't feel confident about taking up higher challenges and don't want to leave their comfort zone. What about you?

"Everything that happens to you is a reflection of what you believe about yourself. We cannot outperform our level of self-esteem. We cannot draw to ourselves more than we think we are worth."

- Iyanla Vanzant

What is Self-esteem?

According to WHO (World Health Organization), a leading cause of illnesses is not diabetes, physical injury or cancer, the leading cause of ill-health and disability throughout the world is depression. According to the Anxiety and Depression Association of America, about 40 million people over the age of 18 suffer from anxiety disorders. Low self-worth and low self-esteem can lead to anxiety and depression. It can lead people to opt out of life and numb out on drugs and alcohol, even attempt suicide because the pain of feeling unworthy is too severe to bear.

As a human being, each individual has a tremendous amount of potential and they can accomplish anything in their life but it requires unleashing the true potential and channelizing our energy in the right direction. Our self-esteem plays a vital role in unleashing our true potential.

Self-esteem is how you feel and think about yourself. It's an internal evaluation of your qualities and attributes. True self-esteem depends on how you value and respect yourself, since its self-esteem, it is all internal. It has nothing to do with what others think of you, it's not about external circumstances, and it has everything to do with the inner game of yours.

Self-esteem is very important in determining the quality of success and happiness in your life. If you have high self-esteem, you accept yourself the way you are, you feel good and confident of doing what you want to do which keeps your energy level up for everything that you do. With high self-esteem, you stop blaming your rejections, mistakes, failures, ill-health and start focusing on your strengths, successes and accomplishments that you have had in your life so far. This continues to motivate you for the future.

People with low self-esteem feel pity, depressed, victim and under-confident for themselves. They don't accept any compliment, judge themselves to be inferior to others and can't unleash their true potential. They usually underestimate themselves, give up on their personal and career goals, don't think that they can boost their performance and accomplish anything significant in their life.

Now the question is, how do you think and feel about yourself? Do you feel worthiness or are in love with yourself? Do you think you can go out and create a life that you want? Do you have a high self-esteem? If yes, you are taking a step further in mastering the art of peak-performance.

How do you evaluate your self-esteem?

Self-esteem is all internal but so often we evaluate our self-esteem through external factors, we seek validation of others to determine how valuable we are, we rely on our friends to praise us to feel good, we rely on 'likes' and 'followers' on social media to make us feel valued, we rely on our education grading system and several other external factors to validate us. We rely on our increments and promotion to make us feel worthy, and for any reason, if we don't get what we expect then we fall into the low self-esteem and don't value ourselves. We become like a doormat, allowing others to walk all over us. Because we allow others to walk all over us, they gladly victimize us and take advantage of us because we are a doormat.

On the other hand, if we have high self-respect then we believe we have the right to be happy and don't need to change ourself for the sake of others.

Causes of low self-esteem and ways to overcome:

Authority figures:

In our life, there are a few authority figures (Parents, teachers and a few more), whom we trust and give them an authority to form an opinion about ourselves. Their opinion becomes so valuable that we start to believe in their opinion about us as a fact. Sometimes we wrongly believe that other people have more insights about us than what we do. If these authority figures have a negative opinion about us, we tend to believe them as fact and suffer from the symptoms of low self-esteem. There are several cases when as a child someone has been commented by their parents or teachers that "they are not good enough", now this statement remains in their mind and they carry this statement even when they enter adulthood due to which they suffer from low self-esteem.

To overcome this negative authority figure, we have to work on our reaction for negative comments that we hear from authority figures. For every negative comment we hear from them about us we have to fight back with positive comments in our mind. We can't stop others what to think about us but it's entirely up to us on how to react for comments like such.

Comparison:

This is one of the easiest ways to feel low self-esteem. If we look at our own history, our parents keep comparing our educational performance with others and we continue to do this while we enter adulthood. The way we currently use social media for comparing ourselves with others is even more dangerous because people only show the best of them on social media and we believe that this is what they are and starting feeling awful for ourselves.

What we have to realize is every individual is unique and has some other skills wherein they are good at. The more we compare ourselves, the more we will feel awful. The best solution is to stop comparing yourself with others but if you can't, remember, that you are not seeing the complete reality, you are only seeing what others want you to see. Think about what you post on social media or tell your friends about yourself. Rarely the failures, right? Usually, people only show off the best part of their life and rarely have the courage to show bad experiences or failures. The best strategy is to feel happy about others without feeling bad about yourself.

Past Mistakes:

Mistakes and choices made in the past, sometimes these mistakes makes you feel bad about yourself and if you continue to think about them and blame yourself for doing those mistakes, you are trapped under low self-esteem.

To overcome this guilt what we have to remember is mistakes, rejections and failures are a part of life. What you can learn from mistakes, you can't learn from success. Think about positive aspects, what you learn from these mistakes and how it can help you in the future. Sometimes one mistake can help you shape your life to an entirely different direction that would have not been possible otherwise. Live a guilt-free life, accept your mistakes and move on instead of continuing to be in guilt about the choices you made.

Negative thinking pattern:

Thoughts and feeling work in the same way most of the time. If you constantly harbor negative thoughts and say negative things about yourself then you continue to feel the same way. An inaccurate thought pattern can lead to an inaccurate feeling pattern.

To overcome this, continue to monitor your thought pattern and challenge your negative thoughts more often. Start doubting your negative thoughts and change your thought pattern gradually to make you feel better. Changing thought pattern from negative to positive works like magic and can significantly help you shift from low self-esteem to high self-esteem.

Negative surroundings:

Negative surroundings severely influence how you think and feel about yourselves. Sometimes your peers make deliberate attempts to pull you down, bullying you or want you to do something that you are not comfortable doing. All these acts are very damaging, it make you feel something is wrong with you and you tend to doubt yourself.

To overcome this, change your surroundings if possible and start surrounding yourself with people who are your well-wishers and help you grow as a human being. You need to have friends who value you and help you maintain a healthy level of self-esteem If it's not possible to change your surroundings then change the way you react to these situations to have a least negative impact on your self-esteem.

Unrealistic Expectations:

Sometimes we have unrealistic expectations from ourselves, this happens due to social pressures or we being over ambitions and expect too much from ourselves. This usually happens with various students who are carrying a burden of grades imposed by their parents, with corporate employees to meet the unrealistic deadline due to pressure by their client and with any human being for achieving any social status due to their family pressure. The failure to meet unrealistic expectations leads to the feeling that you are a failure in general.

To overcome this, it's advisable to have stretched goals but not beyond a level that seems unrealistic. Assess yourself and march towards your goal to make yourself feel the sense of accomplishment. Celebrate small victories to continue to make you feel better. When you celebrate small successes, you give a message to your subconscious that you are doing something that's worth celebrating.

The above causes of low self-esteem are the most common causes and there can be several others but if you can control your thinking pattern and have a strong belief system, it can help you overcome those and have high self-esteem.

What to remember when you have low self-esteem?

1) You are a miracle! Given the odds calculated by the scientists show that you are not born by accident, the odds of you being born are at least 1 to 4 trillion. Therefore, be true to yourself, there is no one like you, so, be humble, be grateful and continue to worth yourself.

2) You are a product of your thinking pattern and belief system; change your thoughts and beliefs to change your life. (Discussed in chapter-3 & 4)

3) Be in a resourceful state to conquer the world. (Discussed in chapter-6)

4) You are a unique individual with own set of strength and weaknesses, focus on your strengths and don't ever compare yourself with others.

5) You can't change how others see you or treat you but you can choose how to feel about yourself and you can also choose to be surrounded by more positive people.

6) Positive inner self-talk is the key to improve self-esteem.

7) Forgive yourself for any bad choices made in the past, don't blame yourself for any reason.

8) Identify your competencies and develop them. If you are a good dancer, focus on this strength rather than brooding over why you can't be a good pianist.

9) Accept compliments, there is a reason someone appreciates you. Take those positively.

Long story short, improving self-esteem is must, and requires a bit of inner work as it involves developing inner habits to continue to feel valued, the more you work on those inner habits the more you think and feel better about yourself. Remember, it can't be done overnight it's a continuous process but you will certainly notice positive changes gradually as you start working on your inner habits. After a reasonable period of your efforts on your inner habits, you will feel calm, compose, confident and start valuing yourself. All these changes help you unleash your potential, career progression, better financial growth and jack-up your performance in various areas of your life.

"Self-esteem is as important to our well-being as legs are to a table. It is essential for physical and mental health and for happiness."

- Louise Hart

Chapter 8

CHANGE THE CHANNEL!

How long you can watch the TV show if you don't like at all? Well! With 100s of exciting and entertaining channels why you will continue to be stuck on the show that you don't like at all? I'm sure you will take the remote and flip the channel immediately, isn't it? You can apply the same strategy when your painful past is being pictured in your mind unexpectedly. Change the channel, start accessing the positive and most wonderful moments to gain strength.

If you are not been able to perform up to your potential for some or other reason doesn't mean that you can't do it in the future. Analyze what went wrong, change your strategy and do it again. You may have deep scars from your emotional wounds of past but take charge immediately, don't let your past determine your future. Your future doesn't have any correlation with your past but yes what you do today will certainly have an impact on your future.

Let go

Let go of painful experiences and failures of past, forgive people who did wrong with you, forgive yourself for all the mistakes that you did and caused you pain and hurt. Change the channel and focus on various positives and good things around you.

If something bad and negative happened to you in the past don't even think about it. Don't talk about that with your friends over and again. Remember, unless you let go of the old negatives, you can't get the new positives.

Every person has good and bad experiences. Good experiences cover our victories, accomplishments and all the events that make us feel good. Whereas bad experiences cover pains, hurts of the past and all negative events that make us feel awful. If you want to be free and stay happy, unshackle yourself from all the bad experiences and keep your mind focus on good things.

Control the controllable:

Ask yourself a question, "Do you want to feel good or want to feel sorry for your negative past?" Your negative past is something where you don't have any control, you can't go back and change that but you are completely in charge of your present. So if you want to be happy, if you want to be free, get the junk out of your mind, stop holding on to it. Don't allow the root of bitterness continue to poison your life. The simple mantra is change the channel, move on and see the magic happens in your life.

Chapter 9

SIMPLE YET AMAZING FORMULA FOR PEAK PERFORMANCE

Simple Yet Amazing formula for peak performance

Performance= Potential-Interference.

This excellent concept has been shared by W. Timothy Gallwey in one of his books 'Inner Game of Tennis'. According to this concept, your performance is equal to your potential if you remove all the interferences. Isn't it simple yet amazing? If you remove your interferences you can perform to your fullest potential and that's what peak performance is.

When we talk about Potential, each one of us, and I repeat it again, each one of us is limitless in terms of what we can accomplish and achieve, we all have limitless potential within us. When we have the desire to make something happen for ourselves or for our businesses, we really find ways to make it happen. If the potential within us is great then what stops us to achieve to what we are capable of? What is holding us back?

Think about how incredible it's to have our performance match with our potential, this is what peak performance level is, but in most of the cases we stay away for this incredible match. Do you know why?

All of us desire to perform up to our potential but we face different forms of interferences from multiple sources that are creating roadblocks to make us perform as per our potential. 'Interferences' are the core reasons we are not been able to perform at our peak potential and these interferences can be due to various external sources or through our internal emotions. We can't be living to our fullest potential unless we minimize or eliminate (if possible) all the interferences that are coming in our way.

Do you think our performance can match our potential if we remove all the possible interferences or there is something else too? We feel motivation and the environment also plays a big role in getting the best out of anyone. The motivation-drive of any individual determines how enthusiastic an individual is towards his goal. A motivated individual with no interferences can do wonders if the person gets the right environment. So here's the extended formula for performance:

Performance = (Potential- Interference) x Motivation x Environment

In the upcoming sections, we will go over possible interferences in greater detail. We have already gone through the fixed mindset, limiting beliefs and low self-esteem that are the biggest interferences but apart from those there are a few more possible interferences that are holding us back and not letting us perform up to our potential. Here are some of those:

#1. Skills:

There are various studies that suggest skills can be one of the top most hindrance to hold us back from performing with our maximum potential but the good thing is, even if we are not born talented, skills can be cultivated through learning and deliberate practice.

Developing any skill through 4-stage learning process:

One of the key components for peak performance is your skill that serves you to be at your best in your field. Learning any skills requires consistent efforts, practice and patience, Abraham's Maslow's 4 stages of learning gives us valuable insights on how we learn anything:

1. **Unconscious Incompetence- 'We don't know what we don't know'**

This is a stage in which we are completely ignorant about our incompetence or deficiencies and 'we don't know, what we don't know'. We stay confident because we are ignorant about our incompetence.

Example: Most of the corporate professionals who are not getting intensive feedback about their skills come under this stage of unconscious incompetence.

2. **Conscious Incompetence- 'We know that we don't know'**

"Wisdom is knowing what you don't know."

- Socrates

Under this stage, we grow our awareness and realize the areas where we are not competent enough. As we learn about our incompetence and extent to which we are incompetent, our confidence drops and we feel uncomfortable.

At the same time, we also realize the importance of improving those skills and we also realize that once those incompetencies will improve, we will improve our productivity and effectiveness. With this learning, we commit ourselves, to put our hard work to learn and practice new skills so we can move on to the next stage which is 'Conscious competence'.

Example- A recently promoted manager, after his few failures in delivering speeches to his team, realizes the skills where he is not good at.

3. Conscious competence- 'We work at what we don't know'

Under this stage, we achieve 'conscious competence' with our committed efforts and we can perform the skill but it takes effort and work. As we know how much we learn and start performing without much assistance, our confidence increases but we are still in a stage where we are consciously performing that skill.

Example- The same manager after learning and practicing, started producing much better but he is quite conscious and still not at his best but nonetheless, it has increased his confidence and he is doing what he couldn't do earlier.

4. Unconscious competence- 'We don't have to think about knowing it'

This is the stage when skill becomes your habit and enters in the subconscious part of mind. In this stage, your confidence is at peak and you no longer have to remember what you have to concentrate on what you know/do. This is where we can do something effortlessly.

Example: The same manager is effortlessly delivering what he is expected and no longer has to be conscious as it has entered into the automaticity.

These 4 stages of learnings can be applied to any area of life: dancing, singing, painting, parenting, and meditating, professional learning and so on. In order to be most productive and perform at peak, your goal is to realize 'unconscious competence' and that's where magic starts happening. Everyone can embrace the state of unconscious learning and perform at peak as it's available to all.

#2. Excuses

Do you 'make excuses' to be excused from the task or any responsibility? Excuses are no less than a terrorist to our peak potential. While some of the excuses are legitimate but most of the excuses are illogical and stupid reasons to defend ourselves for avoid doing things that are essential and critical to achieve our goals. Oh yes, to make it look good to you, you may toss some legitimate and valid reason for not doing certain things that are mandatory. I have heard people using these phrases to justify themselves:

You don't understand, I had to do 'X' just because of...

If you understand why we did 'X' then you would appreciate...

I couldn't do 'X' because it was raining in the morning.

I got late to the office because I couldn't get up on time.

Are you allowing these sort of reasons to interfere in achieving what you want to achieve? And, if you are then you are compromising with your values and performance and selling your potential short. To the extent, you are allowing excuses not to interfere in your way you are progressing towards performing at your peak.

Here's how you can blow out your excuse-making pattern and enhance your performance:

1) Quality-check of your Excuse:

When you plan to take action on elevating your performance, installing any new habit for success or accomplish any goal what type of excuses emerge in your mind? What's the quality of your excuses? Is it just an excuse? Does it enhance your performance or empowers you? How are you going to accomplish your goal if you continue with that excuse?

2) Blowing out your excuses with 'No' state:

After the quality check of your excuse, access your strong 'No' state for your excuses and ask these strong questions to move forward:

Does this excuse serve your purpose and goal?

Are you going to let this excuse hold you back?

Is this excuse bigger than your goal?

3) Effect of excuse blow-out:

After the excuse blow-out, how do you feel now? What comes to your mind? Most likely you will realize that overcoming excuses is essential to move forward in your life and help you match your performance with potential.

Thus the conclusion is, be stronger than your strongest excuse, perform optimally and success is bound to come your way.

"Maturity is when you stop complaining and making excuses, and start making changes."

- Roy T. Bennett

#3. Fear

You know what it takes to be a peak performer, you know what habits and circle you have to be surrounded with to excel in your performance, you know what steps are mandatory for self-mastery, but when it comes to taking action, executing those strategies and installing new habits you are crippled by the phrase 'What if'. This is nothing but your most inhibiting internal emotions called 'Fear'. It keeps you away from limitless opportunities that surround you and puts you in a defensive position. While some of the fears may have some basis but many of our fears are baseless.

"Fear only become powerful, when you give it your power."

- Robin Sharma

By default, our mind tries to keep us safe but in the process it keeps us away from the challenging opportunities that can take us towards success. If we can win the battle with our own 'Fear', we can conquer the world and come up like a Steller performer. In fact, some of our fears are unrealistic but because we give them too much significance and meaning and listen to them more frequently. It can get in our way and barricade us for performing at our best.

Crippled by Fear?

Do you have any fear that is creating interference on your way to success? How are those fears impacting you? Identify those fears, is it the fear of failure, fear of the unknown or any other fear as most of the fears kill our creativity and move us away from taking risks. While in fear, we only look at what can go wrong and that's not the state to bring innovation and peak performance. It's mandatory to get rid of your unrealistic and unproductive fears but the question is how.

Fear blow-out; but how?

To overcome your unrealistic and unproductive fears, you should identify what are you fearful about. To what extent it's dangerous? Do you have resources of talent, knowledge and confidence to negate the effect of fear? Continue to question and challenge your fear, anticipate the worst-case scenario for taking that action and doing it no matter what. Being status-quo is not going to help you reach the level where you want to be.

Stop imagining all the things that could go wrong and start now. Always remember, fear is just an anticipation of pain and it's not real pain. Those who are successful also confronted fear but they took the action despite the fear and they reached where they wanted to. They knew, being in fear and not taking any action will not take them where they want to go. What about you? A simple formula to overcome fear is, feel the fear and do it anyway.

"Don't allow your fear to come in your way. If you want to get something you have never got, you have to do something that you have never done."

Make your goals bigger than your fears and move on! Your motivational drive to goal can't be small enough to hold you back. When you face the fear you become fearless and the same fear will never hold you back. Feel the fear and do it anyway!

"Fear is the pathway to become fearless."

#4. Procrastination:

"Procrastination is one of the most common and deadliest of diseases and its toll on success and happiness is heavy."

- Wayne Gretzky

What's the first thing you do when your alarm rings in the morning? I am sure you don't walk your fingers to the snooze button. Oh...you do! Why do you press the snooze button and don't wake up on the time that you set up last night in your alarm? Are you suffering from the disease of procrastination? If yes, do you know the consequences? It will keep delaying you from taking any action and the delay in action will also be delaying you accomplishing your goal.

YOLO! Yes! You Only Live Once and thus stop procrastinating as it has the potential to not only make you realize your optimum potential and reach the zenith of your peak performance but also leads you to your goals and objectives thereby giving you a perfect sense of satisfaction in life.

Here's the practical way out to beat your procrastination to get things done:

1) Write your goals:

Writing your goals every day in your morning journal will keep reminding you about those goals and motivating you to beat your procrastination. Set challenging yet achievable goals, if goals are not achievable, procrastination snakes in.

2) Pain Vs Pleasure theory:

One of the most obvious reasons behind procrastination is the hard work involved, Start taking baby steps and once you start succeeding in those endeavors you stay on the top.

For example, you delaying to start exercising as you are scared that you will have to continue exercising and for that, you need to take a pain of waking up half an hour early. However, once you start exercising for a few days and getting good results the pleasure of being in good health looks more than the pain you are taking.

3) 21 Days Procrastination Diet:

It's easier said than done but it's a game-changer, so it's worth trying. Stay on procrastination diet for 21 days and pick one thing each day that you have been resisting on for the past some time. It could be as simple as getting up at 6:00 AM on day 1. If you are procrastinating morning walk, go to a morning walk on day 2. This way you can write down 21 things for each day that you have been procrastinating but doing it now.

As you start doing things that you have been procrastinating, you are rewiring the way your brain works and you build more willpower to beat the procrastination.

4) Either you succeed or learn:

If the fear of failure leads you to procrastinate, remember, it is always better to try and learn than not trying at all. Also always remember Failures teach you several precious lessons and take you one step closer to success when you perform optimally and persevere irrespective of the results.

5) Distraction-Free environment:

Distraction-free environment is mandatory to beat procrastination. Any kind of distractions will encourage you to procrastinate. For example, if your Facebook notifications and Twitter notifications keep buzzing while you are working on your most important goal, what will you do? You will check those notifications and you will delay and procrastinate your most important mission.

"Procrastination is like a credit card: it's a lot of fun until you get the bill."

- Christopher Parker

Chapter 10

GET ANYTHING YOU WANT...AN OUTCOME-DRIVEN APPROACH

Do you wonder how few people get what they want whereas others struggle to get even closer to their deepest desire? Are you one of them, who is living to pay bills and survive? Are you caught up in the trap of making a living rather than designing a life? Researches says, only 3% of adults write their goal. Have you written your goal yet? If yes, well done! You are already among the 3% of people for which you deserve a pat on your back... but if not, it's your chance to be in the top 3%.

"Setting goal is the first step in turning the invisible into visible."

- Tony Robbins

One of the key pre-requisite of success in any area of life is to set 'Goals'. Successful people have Goals and those who are not having any goal can rarely be successful. If you want to discover the possibilities within you, you must find a challenging goal to push you beyond your limits and discover your true potential

The fundamental of performing at the peak is setting challenging goals. You can't grow without having a Goal. If you don't have a goal then your life is GOL (Hindi Zero). Set a benchmark and do your Best. Let's be the one whom people treat as a role model. You can do miracles if you have goals.

Endowment-effect of Goal:

When we set a goal for ourselves, we don't just set it, we own it and it becomes a part of us. It also becomes our identity and who we are. In psychology it's called "Endowment-effect", a phrase coined by Richard Thaler, It says when you own something, you are committed to it, you don't want to give it up and it becomes your identity. When we set a goal, we put our entire focus and change our mindset on how to accomplish this.

Why setting goals is the key to success?

"Your goals are the roadmap that guide you and show you what is possible for your life."

- *Les Brown*

Having a challenging goal is the key to unleash your potential and perform at peak, it gives you purpose and direction. It also gives you a concrete endpoint to aim for and get excited about. Goal is what you want to be or what you want to accomplish in the future. It is the utmost motivation that keeps calling you all the time irrespective of how tired you are in your journey. Goal is like an address on an envelope, without which, the envelope can reach nowhere.

In my entire career, I have interacted with thousands of individuals and what I have discovered is, the ones that are having goals are the ones who are highly successful than the ones not having goals. There are a number of success stories of not just individuals but big organizations that are having challenging goals.

In 1960, Honda set a goal and the punch line of their goal has been "we will destroy the competition". After they had this goal, they started brainstorming on how to reach this goal and thought about how good they could become in the process of reaching this goal. Therefore, once you set the goal, your brain starts thinking about ways on how to accomplish this.

In 1970, Nike set a goal; "Crush Adidas". Do you think these goals are easy? Well, It's not! But once you decide goals like such, you will continue to have sensation in your mind and you will start exploring various ideas on how to achieve this goal.

If you are a student, set a goal of topping the upcoming competitive exams and surpass the grades of Steller performers of earlier years.

If you are a business owner, set a goal that you feel is challenging which can be in terms of revenue or being a leader in your industry.

If you are an individual performer, set a goal of reaching to next level in your career path.

Don't have a goal yet? Make One! Set a challenging goal and drive your actions towards that goal. There is no point being directionless and running without any endpoint in mind.

10 Key components of goals

#1. Clarity:

Having absolute clarity about your goal is extremely important. Let's be crystal clear about what you want. Albert Einstein said, "Your goal must be so clear that a 6 year child could understand it so clearly and explain to another 6-year-old child and be able to tell you if you would achieve your goal or how close you were." The goal has to be extremely clear, specific and measurable.

#2. Reason:

"Reason comes first, action comes later."

As a child, you were very curious to ask 'Why' for almost everything around but as you grow into an adult, your curiosity diminishes. Knowing 'Why' is very important to help you understand yourself and various things around you.

Find out why it's important for you to achieve the goal. 'Why' gives you a compelling reason for doing 'what you are doing'. Knowing 'why you do what you do' for the goal fires you inside out that drives you all the way to go for it. When you know your 'Why' figuring out 'how' is not a big deal. Having a strong 'Why' for your goals is one of the key components for having them achieved. Your 'Why' has to be bigger than the fears, excuses and obstacles that you face on your way to achieve your goal. Make your 'Why' strong as your life is dependent on that.

The more compelling your why is, the more motivated you will be to accomplish your goal. Build a strong emotional connection with your goal and you will see the obstacles and interferences are no more hindrance on your way to achieve that goal.

#3. Trust:

Don't create a seed of doubt in your mind for the goal that you set. Have faith in your potential and trust the process. You can't go half-heartedly and see yourself reaching your goal. You have to build a relationship of trust with your goal and give your best to see yourself reaching your goal.

#4. Price:

What is the price you are willing to pay to accomplish this goal? Every goal requires efforts, the bigger the goal, the bigger the efforts. What sacrifices are you willing to make to accomplish the goal? For example; if your goal is to stay fit and lose weight, are you willing to pay the price of getting up early in the morning, hitting the gym for a few hours and adhering to the diet recommendation consistently until you achieve your goal?

#5. Strategize:

Strategize on how you will proceed further and work towards the goal. Think about what are the resources (money, skills and professional help) that you need. Take a piece of paper and describe in detail what are the skills, abilities, attitudes and beliefs that you would need to develop in order to achieve your goals and start making plans of having them when you need them.

#6. Obstacles:

Think about possible obstacles that can hold you back from achieving your goal. To identify the possible obstacles, ask yourself why have you not achieved your goal already? And you will get a bunch of possible obstacles that were the bottleneck in achieving your goal. Once you have the list of obstacles, plan on how to deal with them to stay unshaken towards the final goal. You can apply the 80/20 rule which I have shared in chapter 12. Evidentally, 80% of the obstacles that hold you back are inside yourself and only 20% are outside.

#7. Breakdown the timeline:

Breakdown your goal into various small milestones and set timeline for each milestone. These milestones can further be divided into weekly or daily actionable steps. Remember, the smaller your actionable steps, the more your mind can believe in achieving them and that confidence plays a huge role. Setting timeline also helps in monitoring the progress and expelling procrastination.

#8. Declare:

Publically declare your goal to continue getting driven towards your goal. When you publically declare your goal, you will find it more difficult to stray from your path when challenges set in. When the road to your goal gets a little bumpy, your public announcement may keep you going or your loved ones will assist you to carry on with your goal. Once you declare the goal, you almost set yourself up for not giving up and that makes things happen.

#9. Action:

The journey of 10,000 steps starts with the first step! Figure out what is the first step that you have to take to start working on your goal and take that action. Take tiny steps to start before you take the epic action! And Yes, Consistent action! No one wants to hear, what you say, you are going to do, everyone wants to see you executing. Do something every day that takes you closer to what you want to accomplish. Talk less, do more is the mantra! Don't just talk, let's do what it takes to be a genius!

#10. Make it real:

Once you have already figured out the 9 components of goal that are mentioned, it's time to make it real before it converts into reality. Remember, your subconscious mind has 90% power and it doesn't know the difference between reality and imagination. To ensure the attainment of your goal, you must condition your subconscious mind in advance to feel the pleasure as if you have already attained the goal. At least once a day, you must emotionally connect with your goal and enjoy the experience of achieving it. Think about how would you feel about yourself. How your life will change? What people will say to you? This will create a neural pathway between where you are and where you want to go. Not just that, this intense conditioning will allow you to attract the required resources and to take the most effective action.

So, what are you waiting for Start now! There are a bunch of goal setting approaches shared in this chapter ahead!

Approaches to Goal Setting:

Given the importance of having a goal, there are various experts who have jumped in and shared their expertise on how the goal is to be created. Here are some of those goal-setting approaches that you can follow:

1) S.M.A.R.T.

2) S.M.A.R.T.E.R. (NLP Model)

3) H.A.R.D

4) WOOP

5) B.H.A.G

SMART

This is one of the most common and traditional methods of goal-setting. This became famous when Jack Welch, one of the most successful CEOs, inducted this goal-setting model in General Electronics in the early 1980s. Acronym for SMART is Specific, Measurable, Achievable, Relevant, Time bounded.

S-Specific: Be specific and clear about what you want.

M-Measurable: How are you going to measure the progress and accomplish the milestones?

A-Achievable/Actionable: Your goal should be achievable. If you feel it's not achievable, your mind won't encourage you to put efforts into trying to achieve it. Does it have a clear Action plan?

R-Relevant: For personal goal-setting, this means creating a goal that gets you where you want to be in life. Take it back to developing a goal that's exactly what you want. It's important to do this right.

T-Time bounded: This is critical to achieving a goal. Without setting a time of when you want to achieve it, you allow yourself to procrastinate. With an exact date, you are locked in.

With time and experience, various experts have realized that the definition of SMART acronym needs to be updated to make it more effective.

HARD GOALS

The concept of HARD Goals has been developed by Mark Murphy, Bestselling author of 'Hundred Percenters', in his book 'Hard Goals' and it stands for:

H-Heartfelt: Developing a strong emotional connection to your goal at intrinsic, personal and extrinsic levels so you are motivated to put your power behind the goal and make it happen for you.

A-Animated: Visualizing the goal is very powerful. Create a picture in your mind about how you would feel or how the world will look at you after you achieve your goal. Have a stronger image of your goal as if the goal has been achieved and see the miracles of seeing it happen in reality with your massive action.

R-Required: Convince yourself that this goal is absolutely necessary for your overall success and not optional anymore. Procrastinating this may have a severe adverse effect on your overall career.

D-Difficult: Your goal should be challenging enough to unleash your potential. Setting an easy goal will continue to keep you in the comfort zone. Set goals that push you to perform at a level higher than what you have done earlier. While setting the goal, you shouldn't set the goal that is quite easy and can be achieved within the comfort zone. However, it shouldn't be physically impossible as well, else you will give up without even trying. You should aim for the 'Sweet Spot' which is just above the 'comfort zone' and below the 'physically impossible' level.

Remember the words of Mr. Azim Premji while setting your goal, "If people are not laughing at your goal, your goals are too small."

SMARTER

NLP goal-setting model (well-Formed outcome model) is the one that is formulated in a way that significantly increases the chances of the goal being achieved for its inherent characteristics. It allows us to condition our mind to drive us towards the goal. The standard S.M.A.R.T approach is extended to S.M.A.R.T.E.R to make it more effective. Our brain primarily works from our sensory system (Sound, Picture, feelings) and the NLP goal-setting model helps us in making our goal sensory specific. NLP model of goal setting also ensures that our unconscious mind and energy are aligned to our goal in achieving it.

It's my humble request to approach the SMARTER model with an open mind to make it more effective:

S- Specific & Simple

Specific: Goal has to be very specific and clear. Instead of saying "I want to make more money" or "I want to lose weight" be specific and say "I want to make 2 Lakhs per month" or "I want to lose 10 kg". Quantifying the goal gives a clear target to our mind that our mind, hence makes our mind work for the goal.

Also, it let's add the element that is sensory-specific to your goal for example, what you will be seeing, feeling and hearing when you will achieve your goal.

Simple: Goal has to be simple to understand; doesn't mean that it should be simple to achieve. We usually have the tendency to delete, distort or generalize if the goal not simple.

M-Measurable, Meaningful, Motivating, More than one way to achieve it:

Measurable: Goal has to be measurable and adding numbers and amount to the goal makes it measurable without which it's almost impossible.

Meaningful & Motivating: Goal has to be meaningful so you continue to get motivated towards the goal. While setting the goal ask a question to yourself "How motivated you will be after you accomplish the goal?"

More than one way to achieve it: If your goal has more than one way to achieve then it gives you the choices and you can choose the one that suits you the most.

A-Achievable, All areas of life, as if now.

Goal should be challenging yet achievable. While setting the goal you must set the goal that stretches you beyond your comfort zone but you must continue to believe that it's achievable. If you feel it's not achievable then your mind won't encourage you to put in efforts to achieve it. While setting a challenging yet achievable goal, you can also take the reference of someone who has achieved a similar goal in a broadly similar situation. Set your goal slightly higher to surpass what has already been achieved.

All areas of life: Your goal should positively impact all the areas of your life. If it can't impact positively then it shouldn't have any significant negative impact in other areas of your life. This will make sure you are maintaining the work-life balance. Ask yourself a question, "What's the impact of your goal on all areas of your life?"

As if now: See your goal as if it's happening now or it has already happened. Visualization is very powerful. Have a stronger image of your goal as if the goal has been achieved and see the miracles of seeing it happen in reality with your massive action.

Action: Action is one of the most critical aspects to accomplish your goal. Create a list of the key action that you are required to take in order to accomplish your goal. Remember "Action brings result".

R- Realistic

The goal you set has to be realistic. There is a very thin line between 'Realistic' and 'Achievable'. A goal may be achievable but sometime it may not be realistic. You have to make sure it has to be realistic as well as achievable.

For example; your goal is to make 10 Million in the first year of your business. Is it achievable? Yes, anything is possible, yet it looks unrealistic.

T-Timed, Towards:

Timed: Your goal achievement should have a specified date and time (if possible). For example, Instead of setting a goal of losing 10 Kg of weight within 6 months we must set a goal of losing weight by 31st December 2020.

Towards- We all know our thoughts become our reality so your goal should clearly state what you want, instead of what you don't want.

E- Ecology

Ecology is the consequence of you achieving your goal. The goal you are setting must be right for you, people around you and for society in general. It should not have any negative consequences on any of these. While setting a goal, ask yourself a question, "What will happen when you achieve the goal?" If the consequence of you achieving the goal is not ecological, you must adjust your goal.

R- Resources:

What resources (Time, Money or Skills) are required to accomplish those? Do you already have all of these? If not, how you will arrange the required resources? Create a proper plan and start taking action in this direction.

Example of Smarter Goal: Wow! It is 31st March 2020 and I'm happily celebrating the launch of my first book 'the genius you', with my friends, family and business network. I am feeling extremely excited to present the first copy of my book to my Mom.

WOOP

WOOP is yet another goal-setting strategy, created by Gabriele Oettingen with his colleague after 20+ years of scientific research. Oettingen introduced this strategy in 2014 in her book 'Rethinking Positive Thinking'. WOOP stands for Wish, Outcome, Obstacles, and Plan. It is based on the science of 'Mental Contrasting' and can be effectively used for all the areas of behavior change including excellence at work.

Steps to set your goals thru WOOP:

W-Wish: Wish something that you would like to accomplish in real life. It could be your big career goal or a small personal goal. Make sure it's dear to you, exciting and challenging enough but realistically possible to achieve by the set due date.

O-Outcome: Imagine the best outcome of your goal and comparing it with where you are now. Think about how you will feel after your goal is accomplished. Create as clear picture as possible. Output has to be truly fulfilling.

O-Obstacles: Think about your personal obstacles that hold you back from accomplishing your goal. Think deeply, are your inner obstacles stopping you? Take enough time to imagine all your main obstacles.

P-Plan: Create an effective action plan on how you will overcome the obstacles that you have identified. Create 'if (Obstacles) then (action)' statement to overcome your obstacles. If 'X' obstacle happens then you will take 'Y' action. Create a list of the action plans for all the obstacles so you know what to do if any of the obstacles arise.

One of the most important parts of WOOP goals is imagining the end result with feeling as well as imagining all the probable obstacles with an action plan. In her book, Oettingen mentioned that being positive is very good but mere positive thinking may not get you anywhere but WOOP can. She has also developed a mobile app that allows the user to set goals.

Are you ready to WOOP it out?

BHAG (Big Hairy Audacious Goal)

BHAG (pronounced as Bee hag), Big Hairy Audacious Goal, is a term invented by Jim Collins and Jerry Porras in one of their most popular books, 'Good to Great'. BHAG is your visionary goal to be achieved in 10-25 years. Having a personal BHAG helps you move towards your clearly defined long term goal.

How to build your personal BHAG:

1) BHAG should not be unrealistic and should be based on deep understanding.
2) While building your BHAG, you should take consideration of:
    a. What you are deeply passionate about
    b. What drives your economic logic

c. What you are best at (Your differentiator)

3) It should be for a long period; 10-25 Years.
4) It should be clear and compelling.
5) It reflects your core value and purpose.
6) It should have a start and end date.
7) Goal should be quantitative so we can measure and qualitative and can emotionally connect to it.
8) We should share this with others to feel ourselves accountable.

Which goal-setting approach is better?

SMART or HARD?

The purpose of setting goals is to have a clear direction so we can take the appropriate action to accomplish them. Both SMART and HARD to some extent serve the purpose. SMART goals are very simple and help in clearly mapping out a plan to achieve them. Whereas HARD GOALS are visualizing the path to Goal. A smart goal to some extent makes us believe that we can only think about the goal that is achievable whereas HARD goals make people even more courageous and they go after the bigger goals. Hard goals also encourage us to associate feeling and emotions with our goal which sometimes is a great driving force.

SMART or WOOP?

SMART goals, theoretically, seem catchy but it's not inspiring as it's not challenging whereas WOOP allows to set difficult goal to push our limits. Unlike WOOP, SMART leaves not much room for creativity. WOOP also uses imagination to our end-goal whereas SMART goal doesn't have any imagination to keep us excited.

SMART or SMARTER?

'SMARTER', an NLP based goal setting model is quite effective, it not just about pushing ourself for a challenging goal but also adding 'As if now' factor through which we can add the feeling and emotions of accomplishing our goal. It also checks for ecology, available resources and most importantly it checks to have our goal sensory-specific.

Based on the research by various experts, most of the goal-setting model serve the purpose if those are very well supported by feedback mechanism and massive action. Which type of goal-setting approach to go for, depends on individual's choice. All we have to make sure is we must follow one of those models that pushes our limits, gives us direction, keeps us motivated for the goal that we are emotionally attached with.

Think it and Ink it:

Writing goals is 10 times more effective, write your goals and put them at a place where you can see them more frequently. Let your goals reach your subconscious mind as many times in a day as possible. Keep a goal card in your pocket. Set your Mobile and laptop screen with your goals to keep reminding you all the time. While inking them, make sure you bifurcate short term, long term and life goals with specific dates. Also mention a few quick action items for each goal so you are in action mode and know what to do.

"People with clear, written goals, accomplish far more in a shorter period of time than people without them could never Imagine."

- Brian Tracy

How to set and achieve any goal in real life:

1) Write 5 goals for each area of your life (personal, professional, career/business, health, relationship, etc.) that you would like to accomplish in the next 6 months. Don't restrict your imagination, be like a kid and have as bigger goals as you can think of.
2) Identify the top one goal from each category so you can have your extreme focus on the goals.
3) Identify 3 goals out of the 5 above and these 3 goals will be your most important goals (MIG).
4) For each MIG above, write down why it's important to you? What would you gain by achieving these goals?
5) What's the price you are willing to pay?
6) List out 3 most important skills that are needed for the goal? Do you have those skills? If not, how will you acquire those?
7) List out 3 most important people who will help you achieve this goal?
8) What other resources are required to accomplish your goal?
9) List out top 3 possible obstacles that may come your way? How to get rid of them?

10) List out various milestones and activities to be performed on a daily basis to accomplish your goal, have them in your calendar and take consistent action.

11) Read your goal twice a day and visualize them as if you have achieved your goal.

Chapter 11

EMPOWERING ECOSYSTEM

Change your circle, change your influence!

"You're the average of 5 people you spend most time with."

- Jim Rohn

Influence of surroundings:

There is an old saying, "Show me your friends and I will tell you who you are." While this saying may not be completely true for everyone but to some extent it is true based on the law of average. Environment and people around you make a huge impact on who you are and how well you will do in your life. When you surround yourself with positive and high-performers, chances of you doing so well in your life is much higher, whereas, you suffer a lot if the people in your circle are negative or narrow-minded. The influence of your surroundings has tremendous power to unleash your true potential and push you to perform at your best.

Positive people continues to lift you higher in your life. They will show you all the reasons why you can do. Whereas, your surroundings not being positive continue to hold you back and give you strong reasons why you can't do. People around you influence your behavior, attitude, action and results. Eventually, you start to think and behave like they do.

"According to research by social Psychologist Dr. David McClelland of Harvard, the people you habitually associated with determine as much as 95% of your success or failure in life."

Mirror Neurons:

Mirror neurons are the brain cells that get activated when we see someone doing something. Mirror neurons are essential for imitation which is key for learning process. These group of neurons are activated right from our birth and this is what allows us to learn so many things. It's also important in planning our action and understand the intention behind action.

As a social being, we are programmed to learn from others. Seeing what people are doing around us activates our mirror and it gives us a tangible experience of learning.

Mirror neurons produce emotional contagion, which is a process through which a person or group influences the emotions and emotional behavior of another person or group.

Who do you spend most time with?

Now the question is if you are the average of people you spend most time with, who you are spending most time with? Are they helping you unleash your potential and perform at your best? Are they helping you accomplish your goal? Are they adding any value to your life? Are they happy seeing you successful? Are they better than you? Do they inspire you? Do they push you to do your best?

Closely observe your circle and if the answer to these questions is 'No' then you have to take immediate action and make sure you find people that can have a positive impact on your life.

Remember, "You can't hang out with negative people and expect positive life."

Which type of people to surround with?

"Surround yourself with the dreamers and the doers, the believers and thinkers, but most of all, surround yourself with those who see the greatness within you, even when you don't see it yourself."

- Edmund Lee

Having positive, inspiring and successful people around can consciously and subconsciously challenge you to be at your best. Spend time with people who inspire you, encourage you to lift your game, motivate you, and perhaps a little higher in scale on where you want to be.

If you want to excel your performance in various areas of your life, surround yourself with people who are ambitious, people who are hunger to learn and grow, people who are pushing you to do your best, people who are adding value to your life, people who are doers and problem-solvers, people who are action-takers, and people who have the mindset of anything could be possible.

Stay away from people who harbor limiting beliefs and fixed mindset, people who say "You are not good enough", and "You Can't do something", people who hold you back, people who are not ambitious, and people who are having average mindset.

If you are the smartest person in your circle, who you will learn from and how you will grow? You must surround yourself with people who are better than you in some way so you can learn from them and grow, people who are having similar goals and are already on the same path that you are.

How surrounding Impacts:

You can't be what you can't see:

Having surrounded with the people who you want to become gives you a lot of exposure. This exposure will help you understand what it takes to be a person like them or having skills like them. You can't be, what you can't see and that's the biggest challenge. Being exposed to unique experiences is really important. When you see them you will continue to get pushed to be like them and that brings out the best in you. If you want to be multi-millionaire, be with them to get an understanding of what it takes to be a multi-millionaire, observe their habits, their beliefs, plan, strategies and action.

Surrounding with right mindset brings the right result:

Having surrounded with positive, inspiring and successful people continue to make you believe that you can also do that. Surrounding with successful people also gives you the blueprint that you have to walk on to be like them and that makes your job easier.

The power of positive people around is quite energetic, inspiring and continue to stretch you from your comfort zone and that's where you unleash your potential and give your best.

The experience, the push, the motivation, the Blueprint and the guidance that you can get with the people who are your role model or who you want to be is quite unique and you can't get if you are not surrounded by right-minded people.

Surrounding yourself with people who are pursuing similar goals; when I decided to write this book, I networked with one of the groups that has several authors in that group. Some of them were in the process of completing their manuscript whereas some of them were already authors of published books that were already successful. Being surrounded by that group enlightened me with the skills, required energy, motivation and brilliance that was very helpful to get this book published.

How to get rid of people that are not right-minded?

"Surround yourself with people who are only going to lift you higher."

- Oprah Winfrey

If you are looking for awesomeness and greatness in your life, you have to take massive action that takes you there. If your surroundings are not adding value to move you towards greatness then change it! Don't be afraid to lose some of your friends if those are not positive contributors in your life. You will find the new ones and probably the better ones. Like attracts like, you will certainly attract people who are as passionate and hungry as you are and that's what is going to help you lift you higher.

Negativity is one of the most dangerous diseases, it's like having a virus in your computer and no computer can perform efficiently unless the virus is completely removed. Here's how you can get rid of the negativity that is speeded by people around you:

1) Cut the Crap:

Remember, the dream in your heart may be bigger than the environment in which you are. Sometimes you have to get out of that environment to see that dream fulfilled.

Immediately remove the people from your life who are spreading negatively. Now some of those people may be with you for years but there is no point continuing with them if they are not in sync with your growth path and the direction you want to move on to.

If you can't completely cut the people from your life because they are your close family members and friends then limit your exposure with them. Don't spend much time with them or don't even talk to them about your ambition, career, and life goals, etc. because you know talking to them will fill you in with a lot of negativity.

2) Tree-Mindset:

If you have no option to eliminate the negativity created by people around you then you can be like a tree. What tree does is, it inhales the carbon dioxide (which is a poison) grow with that poison and exhale Oxygen (Positivity). Having a tree-mindset is quite magical for you, listen to all the negativity of people around you, becomes a better person and spread positivity for everyone around you.

If you are strong enough and having tree-mindset, you won't be impacted by the negativity around, In fact you will use that negativity to strengthen your positivity and come up with even stronger positive beliefs.

3) Fuel in Positivity:

After following step 1) & 2), you have already eliminated some of the negativity, now it's the time to fuel yourself with some positivity. If you can't find people immediately to have the positivity around, listen to various Audios, YouTube vides, various positive blogs and fill yourself in with positivity.

How to find right-minded people?

Now you must have realized how impactful it is to be surrounded by positive people who are adding values to our life but the question is where to find those people? Finding the right-minded people is not very difficult. Once you identify who you want to be surrounded with, the next step is to find out where these people usually go or what they do. If you want to be around those who are passionate about personal development, you will find these people are very crazy about attending various personal development seminars, conferences and events. Go there and you will find a bunch of them, choose the ones who resonate most with you. Network with them, spend time with them and continue with them if you find them the ones that you want to have in your ecosystem.

What if you don't have anybody in your circle who you want to be in the future? What if you don't have anybody who helps you learn and lift your life higher?

Ideally, it seems quite strange if you can't find that circle but there are cases wherein you stay in smaller towns or areas where you don't find such type of people. If this is the case then you should take advantage of various indirect or remote resources that are available to you. Some of those can be joining online communities that help you learn, reading books that infuse positivity, listening to various podcasts that inspire you to do your best, and watching YouTube videos that keep motivating you to push you to take action and do your best. Spending time with these may not be as effective as it is inperson but all these modes can significantly infuse the positivity that can help you learn, stay positive, excel your performance and keep growing.

Are you adding value to your network?

The group of positive, inspiring and successful people love to have those in their network who can add some value to them. Do you add value to your surroundings? Do you push them and bring out the best in them?

In general, people like people who are like them or they like who they want to be. If you want to attract someone, you have to be someone who they see value in. There has to be one or more areas where you are adding value to them so they love to have you around for their growth. Become more valuable to attract quality people. Keep working on your self-development and you will become more valuable.

For example, if you want to be in the group of talented software engineers and learn from them, you have to be a good enough engineer so that those who want to be with you see some values in some or other way to stay connected with you.

Choice to choose:

You have a choice to choose the people who surrounds you. Be smart and choose them wisely. While choosing the people, choose the ones who are ambitions, doers, action-takers, goal-oriented. Choose people whom you can learn from, Choose the people who challenge you, choose the people who think alike, choose the ones who are smarter than you in some or other way. Being with the ones who are better than you will continue to push you to be at their level and you will be able to unleash your potential and give your best.

Remember this saying while choosing your surroundings "Who you spend time with is who you become."

Exercise:

1) Think about 5 people who you spent most time with?
2) Are those 5 people adding any value to your life?
3) Are you adding value to their's who you hang out with?

Chapter 12

HOW TO DEAL WITH THE RAREST COMMODITY?

"It's not about 'Having' enough time, it's about 'Making' enough time."

- Rachael Bermingham

Time Management & Prioritization:

Time is precious and one of the rarest commodity that each one of us has. Whether you are a taxi driver or owning billion dollar business, your day can't be longer than 24 hours. This makes time management even more important than what we can think of. Those who are mastering the art of time management are the champions of productivity and performing at their peak. They are able to produce quality deliverables within the same schedule whereas others are struggling to make this happen.

More than 80% of individuals admits that they don't know how to prioritize as well as they would like to and they end up compromising the quality for their most important work. How about yourself?

With the growing responsibilities, are you prioritizing your to-dos in the most productive ways? Do you concentrate on the to-dos that are having a higher impact on your results and outcome? Mastering the art of time management is nothing but prioritizing the most critical tasks. Here are some of the tools and techniques that an individual and teams can use to improve the productivity and maximize their performance:

"The key is not to prioritize what's on your schedule, but to schedule your priorities."

- Stephen Covey.

80/20 Rule:

Are you aware of 80/20 rule, the Pareto principle? 80/20 is one of the most effective ways to enhance your productivity and achieve your goal in less time.

What is 80/20 rule for prioritizing?

Most of us tend to assume that inputs and outputs are perfectly balanced, for example, 50% of inputs will always result in 50% of the output in the real world. But according to the 80/20 rule, it says there is a fundamental imbalance between inputs and outputs. In any situation a small % of inputs may produce the majority of the output and majority of the inputs may produce small % of outputs.

80/20 rule was named after its founder, the Italian economist, Vilfredo Pareto back in 1895. 80/20 rule (Pareto principle), which is vital few (or top 20%) and trivial many (or bottom 80%), states that 80% of the results come from 20% of our action and 20% of the results come from 80% of the action.

According to this rule, we are putting most efforts (80%) to some of our to-dos that generates very little (20%) result and putting less efforts (20%) on some of our to-dos that generates more (80%) result. This shows we are not giving enough focus to the to-dos that are most critical.

80/20 rule is just a way to recognize the fundamental imbalance between the input and output, just because it's called 80/20 doesn't mean that the result will always statically be in proportion to 80/20. The imbalance might be 70/30, 90/10 or it can be 60/40 but there will be an imbalance and we have to stay on the top to identify the vital few that produce the majority of the result and focus majority of our resources there.

Does 20% of your efforts give you 80% of the results?

Does 80% of the team completes 20% of the outcome?

How 80/20 rule work in prioritization and Productivity?

According to the 80/20 rule, 20% of the general to-do list will produce a higher impact than the other 80% put together. So, we should focus on those high-impact to-dos that have a greater contribution to the overall results. Here's how you can follow this rule:

Create a list of 10 to-dos, required to perform for that particular project.

Identify the first most important task that has a higher impact than the other 9.

Identify the 2nd most important task that has higher impacts than the others 8.

Now you will realize both these tasks put together have a higher impact than the other 8 to-dos.

Applying this principle we can priorities the higher impact

to-dos and have our most focus on them. The remaining time can be spent on the to-dos that are relatively less impactful in the overall result.

Eat the biggest frog first:

Mark Twain said, "If it's your job to eat a frog, it's best to eat the first thing in the morning. And if it's your job to eat two frogs, it's best to eat the biggest one first."

'Frog' here has been used as a metaphor for difficult and critical to-dos. Starting the day with the most important and critical task is the key. It may seem difficult than the other ones but the reward of completing this is going to have a larger impact than the low-value tasks. The completion of the most critical task gives us the momentum that we can continue to build on for the rest of the tasks.

Identifying the most important is not much difficult, just look at the list of your to-dos and identify which one of them is most important and will have a higher impact on the overall result. Once you identify them, start focusing on them first.

Peak Productive time Zone:

Planning the most critical work around your productivity zone is crucial as well. Find out your peak productive time zone. If your peak productive time zone is morning hours, do most of your critical work in the morning before your energy goes down in the afternoon session. Spend the first 60-120 minutes of your peak productive time zone on the task that is a game-changer and has a higher impact on the result.

The Eisenhower method of prioritization:

It's a matrix-based solution, that divides all the tasks of any given goal or project in 4 quadrants;

Urgent and Important: Tasks that fall under this category require immediate attention. Focus your energy on completing these tasks before you move to the less-sensitive tasks.

Not urgent but important: These are the tasks that are important but can't be postpone to later date. They are not do or die but getting them done is very important.

Urgent but not important: These are the tasks that require immediate attention but are not that important in the overall result so these can be delegated to someone who's competent. The assignee of these tasks must have clear instructions for deliverables.

Not urgent and not important: These are the low priority tasks that can be deleted or done later.

(The Eisenhower Matrix)

	URGENT	**NOT URGENT**
IMPORTANT	**Q1-DO IT NOW** Deadline driven client project Deploy critical bug fix	**Q2-SCHEDULE** Exercise/Meditation Strategic planning
NOT IMPORTANT	**Q3- DELEGATE** Creating weekly report Uploading Bog Post	**Q4-DELETE** Social Media Watching TV

Follow Parkinson's Law:

It states, "Work expands so as to fill the time available for its completion." According to this law, set a tight deadline for any task by assigning less time than it actually requires.

When we reduce the time required to complete the task, we force our brain to focus on the deadline and complete the work within the deadline.

For example, a given task in any project can be completed in 3 days, but when you set the time limit for completing this in 2 days, your brain will get a message to focus and complete this in 2 days and eventually completes this within the deadline.

Multitasking is a strict No...

Juggling several tasks at a time is no more an accepted time management technique in various reputed corporates. As per the studies conducted by various renowned institutions, our brain can only focus one thing at a time and switching between the tasks is no more advisable as it severely impacts the performance and productivity. It takes time to completely shift our thinking from one task to another and ultimately it proves costlier.

Automate:

In the current technology era, there are various tools and techniques available that help in automating various tasks that could have required too much manual effort. Using these tools and techniques is strongly recommended. These tools not just reduce the time required for any task but also improve the productivity. There are various project management tools, communication tools, time tracking tools and several others to make life easier at work. Using these tools is strongly recommended.

To-dos prioritization is one of the key aspects of peak performance for any individual or for a team. By following all these tools and techniques, we can manage our To-dos and prioritize them much better. We can be more productive and focus on the areas that have a higher impact on the final outcome.

"Good things happen when you set your priorities right."

Chapter 13

MODELING A PATHWAY TO EXCELLENCE.

"Success leaves clues. Go figure out, what someone who was successful did, and model it. Improve it, but learn their steps. They have knowledge."

- Tony Robbins.

What's Modeling?

The methodology of recreating and replicating human excellence is called 'modeling' in NLP (Neuro Linguistic Programming). One of the basic underlying assumptions of NLP is, 'If someone in a broadly similar situation can do it, you can also learn and do it'.

NLP has been founded to discover how someone does something excellently so that it could be replicated and taught to others. Bandler, one of the founders of NLP, said that the job of NLP is to create excellence in the performance of human beings no matter what they do.

As a human being, we have tremendous potential to learn any skill through modeling, this is how we have been learning since our childhood. Modeling is the way to reproduce the excellence of others. We can model any human behavior by applying their physiology, thought process and beliefs.

In short, if anyone has produced the result that you want, you can also do the same if you are willing to pay the price that they did. Similarly, if you are excellent in one area and would like to replicate the same in another, you can do so by NLP modeling process.

Modeling involves observing, analyzing the behavior of those doing great and replicating the same in our day to day life.

If you want to be better in your life, maybe a better salesperson, better project manager, better software engineer, better CEO, richer person, better communicator, all you need to do is find a model of excellence, learn how they have been doing and keep doing the way they have been doing.

Advantage of Modeling?

1) Modeling is one of the quickest ways to recreate the excellence that others already have. Modeling helps us learn and replicate excellence that took somebody years to learn and master. Instead of spending our 'Time' in learning those, why not just follow something that somebody has already master after multiple attempts over the years.

2) Modeling excellence leads to improved performance. Modeling, if observed, analyzed and replicated properly, improves the performance of individuals.

3) Individuals that are able to improve their performance through modeling process are able to grow much faster and accomplish their goal in lesser time.

2 ways of modeling excellence:

1) Model-1: This type of modeling relies on watching what the person is doing and copying it. It relies on what you can see and hear.

2) Model-II: This type of modeling involves discovering the internal processes that are happening when a person achieves excellence. So, it discovers not only what the person does but also what values and beliefs the person holds that enables them to achieve excellence.

It investigates the internal mental approaches of the person including strategies Meta programs, neurological levels, timeframes and perceptual positions. It also involves discovering physiology and behavioral patterns found in body language, gestures, eye accessing cues and predicates. For example, if we take supreme athletes you could watch how they run, how they move their bodies, the stance that they have, however, what enables them to win the races time and time again. It has not just to do with the things that you observe on the outside, rather it more of the way they think, their attitude towards running and the strategies that they use to win. That's what makes the difference. Besides, modeling their internal pattern and approach is challenging yet possible.

How to Model?

1) Identify Model:

The first step is to identify the skill or top performer (who has produced consistent results in the same area) that you would like to master. For example, you could model the coding skills of a top software engineer, decision-making skills of any top manager, closure skills of a top salesperson and/or any other skills of any top performer.

Be specific about the skill and context in which you want to use it. Also, define excellence in terms of results that your model of excellence achieves. What you/others see, hear and feel when you have modeled these skills/capabilities?

2) Understand their behavioral pattern unconsciously:

The crux of NLP Modeling is to step into the shoes of your

model and observe their behavioral patterns through repeated imitation. You can observe the following:

- Physiology: Observe their physiology, body movement, breathing pattern, eye movement, Are their heads up or down? Are they standing fully erect or rather compressed?

  Observe their physiology and copy them as it is.

- Intonation: Pay attention to their intonation, vocal behavior, language patter, filters, volume, and pitch.

- Strategy: Every top performer follows a different strategy to excel in doing what they are doing. Observe the key strategies adopted by your model and follow the same strategy.

- Belief system: Those who are outstanding performers have a belief system that helps them unleash their potential and add fuel to their performance. Observe the belief system of your model and understand the consequences of those beliefs in case you model those.

- Others: Few other things to observe to replicate the result of your model:

  - o Values
  - o Energy level
  - o Representation system
  - o Submodality preferences

3) Ask Questions:

If you have an access to your model, you can ask them questions to make yourself aware of your model. Modeling is a process of discovering, so you should become a detective, someone who asks lots of questions and tracks down all the clues to what produces excellence. When your model is imagining using those skills, ask them the questions in the present tense to keep them associated, e.g.

"What are you seeing?" "What are you saying to yourself?" Ask them questions so you understand 'What' and 'How' they do. Keep checking their thinking at each logical level. You can ask them:

- What are your capabilities?
- What is important to you at this time?
- What are you thinking?
- What are you saying and doing?
- How do you connect to other systems?
- Which state you are in?

All these answers will give you a lot of insights that you can replicate in your system for excellence.

4) *Produce result:*

After assimilating the behavior pattern of the top performer, it's time to test your model, while testing you may let go of any element that you feel won't make any difference in the overall result.

5) *Compare the result:*

Do the results you achieve match with the results your model achieves? If they do, you have been successful; if they don't, find the reason for that.

Some Consideration while Modeling:

1) ***Desired outcome:*** It's important to know what you want from the modeling project.

2) ***Available resource:*** NLP Modeling is quite intense as it not just observes the physiology but also observes behavioral patterns which require both time and expertise.

3) ***Finding Experts (Model):*** Finding people who are truly excellent and ready to devote their time to be modeled. This could be challenging sometimes. If you are modeling somebody and you don't have access to the person, you have to rely on most of the information that you can gather through books, videos or articles and that may not produce a similar result.

Modeling is quite effective but it's not something new. Whether in sports, business or any other area, every great performer has modeled the discoveries of others to come up with something exceptional. Every child is modeling the world around them and learning a number of key skills. But the trouble is we are not focused and modeling the way we should be. There are a number of strategies and resources around us that we can model and do wonders but we have to model with extreme focus and not just understand their physiology. We must observe their behavioral patterns to model their excellence. Modeling is such a powerful way to recreate and replicate excellence in performance.

"Success leaves clues, and if you sow the same seeds, you will reap the same reward."

Brad Thor

Chapter 14

POWER-HOUR RITUALS TO DOMINATE YOUR LIFE

"Morning is an important time of day because how you spend your morning can often tell you what kind of day you are going to have."

- Lemony Snicket.

Power-Hour, Kick start your day with energy and positivity.

If you could win the morning you could win the day and one of the surefire ways to be a winner in the morning is to equip yourselves with morning rituals so you don't need to think about what you have to do. When we set up the routine and follow them consistently, especially when we wake up, we create positive momentum for the day ahead. Being genius and world-class performance is less about genetics and talent and more about regular practices, daily routines and habits. It's what you do as a disciplined approach on a daily basis that makes the difference.

The first 60 minutes of morning and last 60 minutes prior to sleep are what I call the 'Power-hour' and 'pre-sleep hour' respectively. How is your routine set up every day? Is your 'power-hour' and pre-sleep hour' set up for the peak performance?

Does your morning usually involves getting out of your bed, taking a quick shower followed by breakfast and start the commute to work? Several people are proud to have a routine like such and they feel good on how quick they are from 'Bed to Desk' but what they don't realize is, in the daily routine like such they don't spend much time with themselves in the morning and march to their workplace without much focus and energy. While they may have a fair bit of success but they have to work very hard for that success and most importantly it may not sustain for a very long time. How about you?

If you go through the morning routine and daily habits of successful people, billionaires, champions and all peak performers, as they get up, they give significant importance to the first 60-90 minutes of their morning routine to boost their energy level. I used to have quite a lazy routine in the morning until the last one year but ever since I have started following the early morning rituals under the guidance of my mentor, my energy and focus has skyrocketed to an entirely different level. I have observed a tremendous amount of uptick in my productivity.

Whether you are a business owner, entrepreneur or senior leader, your morning routine sets the tone for the rest of your day. The first 60 minutes of your morning are very powerful, if you are not energetic and focused during 'power-hour' there is a high probability of you being unfocused and unproductive during your entire day. However, if you have set a routine to start your day strong with energy and focus, the chances of you having a focused, energetic and productive day are much higher.

Consistency is the key:

"We are what we repeatedly do. Therefore, excellence is not an act but a habit."

- Will Durant

Morning routines are part of significant importance for peak performance and there is something magical about repeating the same positive habits every single day. It's not about doing great things occasionally, rather it's doing small things with great commitment consistently that makes the difference. Everyone seems excited forming routines, processes and a protocol but they never stick to it for a long time. However, what differentiates the world-class performers with others is the 'consistency' with which they follow those routines, processes and protocols.

Consistency is the mother of mastery, so if you want to be on the path of self-mastery, be consistent with your 'power-hour' routines and rituals. There are studies conducted on how long it takes to form a habit, some researches say that it takes a minimum of 21 days to form a new habit whereas other researches say it takes 66 days before a new behavior becomes automatic. How long does it take to form a habit varies from habit to habit but it doesn't really matter much. The only way to get to 21st day or 66th is to start with Day 1st and continue to do it until it becomes automatic. It's easier said than done and what you need to remember here is you are running with your older routine for years and it will take some time before your new routine gets into automaticity. So be patient and continue with your new routine to enjoy the benefits once it's into the automated mode.

'Power-hour' Habits:

There are various habits and rituals to pick from but what is important, is to pick the positive habits and routines that work for you and repeat them every day when you get up first in the morning. As you know repetition is the mother of mastery. Here are some of those habits that most successful people engage themselves in for the first 60-90 minutes when they get up every day:

1) **Wake up early:** Waking up early is the most competitive advantage and an important gift that we can give to ourselves because most of our competitors are sleeping at that time. Waking up early is the most important part of daily habits and gives us an edge to practice world-class performance and be at the peak. Time management researcher, Laura Vanderkam, in one of her study, found that 90% of successful executives wake up early in the morning. Going through the routines of many successful people, most of them wake up between 4:00 AM to 6:00 AM. Waking up early gives them a little extra time that they can spend with themselves to energize, organize and plan their entire day. In one of the articles, Christopher Randler, biologist, also states that those who wake up early are proven to be more proactive and handle stress better. Waking up early gives you extra little time for almost everything that you want to do before you head to work and having that extra little time makes you less stressful and calmer than running around for similar things in a hurry.

2) **Digital Detox:** Unplug yourself from your smartphones during your 'power-hour' unless you are using your phones for online courses and podcasts for your morning rituals. Strictly stay away from text messages and emails early in the morning and focus on your self-mastery. Also, check your emails and text message after you complete your power-hour rituals.

3) **Hydrate:** Staying away from dehydration and fatigue is very important. While you are sleeping, you get dehydrate and drinking 2 glass of warm water with organic lemon first thing

in the morning keeps you hydrated and balances your PH level of the body. If you want to be in your most productive state, you should have your brain to be firing on all the cylinders and staying hydrate first thing in the morning boosts your energy level.

4) **Oxygenating exercise:** Our brain is about 2% of our total body weight but it consumes about 20% of oxygen and nutrients, so deep breathing exercise is very important. Oxygenating at the start of the day through deep-breathing exercise is one of the easiest ways to provide the required energy to our mind.

Incorporate 3-5 minutes of deep breathing exercise in your morning rituals whether it is box breathing (focuses on all 4 corners- inhale, breath-hold, exhale, breath-hold), alpha breathing (slow deep breath-inhale through your nose and exhale through your mouth) or any other form breathing exercise that works for you.

If you follow deep-breathing exercise consistently, it will help reduces stress and increase mental clarity, energy and focus.

5) **Workout:** Being committed to health is one of the key ingredients for all the successful people. They all know a healthy mind stays in a healthy body and they give significant importance to their physical health as well. According to several researches, people who exercise regularly are proven to be happier, healthier and more productive.

Do you workout in your daily routine? If not, don't think and make it a part of your everyday regime now, it's a no brainer. A 10 minute quick and intense workout boosts your energy level and keeps your performance level much higher. Morning workout triggers endorphins that increase our brain functioning well by about 37% or more. Morning workouts may include a brisk walk, running, pushups, sit-ups crunches, or any form of exercise that keeps your body physically fit and works well for you.

6) Gratitude :

"Without gratitude and appreciation for what you already have, you'll never know true fulfillment."

- Tony Robbins

Gratitude is one of the most important parts of morning rituals for successful people like Tony Robbins, Oprah Winfrey and several other successful CEOs. Having an attitude of gratitude helps you look at your life positively because if we can't appreciate what we have then we are not going to be given what we really want. Our brain thrives on gratitude, so practicing gratitude as part of your morning rituals helps you set the tone for the rest of the day in a positive direction and overcome negative emotions. When you practice gratitude, it releases dopamine (which contributes to the feeling of pleasure and satisfaction) and serotonin (which contributes to wellbeing and happiness). Both these chemicals make you feel better which will dramatically shift your productivity, focus and energy to a very different level.

Incorporate gratitude in your daily routine, don't take things for granted, be thankful and appreciate what you already have. There are millions of people who don't have shelter for themselves, they face challenges to get food every day, they don't have a support system and friends like you have. Some of them are not even physically fit like you are and they have much bigger life challenges that you can't even think of. Be thankful for even the smallest thing that you have, people who you are connected with, all the situations and circumstances that are helping you directly-indirectly in some or other way. People who include gratitude practice as a part of their morning routine experience more optimism, inspiration, and happiness, as well as better health and more success at work. Having a gratitude board like the vision board is really powerful.

While practicing gratitude:

Be consistent: Choose the number of items you want to be thankful for and be consistent with that format for a long time.

Be specific: Specify why you are grateful for that person, item or event.

Good in the bad: Look for positive outcomes or lessons you learned from negative people, events, items or situations. This will entirely change your perspective towards positivity.

7) **Empowering Affirmation:**

"It's the repetition of affirmations that leads to belief. And once that belief becomes a deep conviction, things begin to happen."

- Muhammad Ali

Affirmations are powerful messages that you want to remind yourself of.

Fill your mind consistently with positive messages to feel empowered during early morning. By reading these messages every single day, you train your mind for success. With enough repetition, these reminders grow into a belief that influences your thoughts and action.

8) Review Goals:

"Review your goals twice every day in order to be focused on achieving them."

- Les Brown

Review your short term and long term goals every day to keep yourself focused, committed and motivated towards your action. While you review your goal, read each goal aloud and think about your actions that can take you closer to your goal. Keep your goals at an easy-to-access place so you continue to get reminded and don't get distracted from your goals.

Reading your goal aloud or writing your goal on a piece of paper (along with a strong reason why you must achieve that goal) will only take about 3-5 minutes but it can do wonders for you. It will automatically change your thinking pattern towards achieving your goal and you will find ways to avoid procrastination.

Visualization of the goal is very powerful, it connects you emotionally with your goal. So, visualize it every day as if you have already achieved your goal. Think about how would you feel about yourself after achieving the goal. How your life will change? What people will say to you? This will create a neural pathway between where you are and where you want to go. Not just that, this intense conditioning will allow you to attract the required resources and to take the most effective action. Remember things happen twice, once in mind and then in your reality. What you sow in your subconscious mind so shall you reap in your reality.

9) **Silence:** Being in silence for 3-5 minutes and observing the flow of breaths is one of the key ingredients for inner growth and nourishment. When you are in silence, you spend time with yourself which refuels your emotional, mental, physical and spiritual self. Being with self keeps you recharged to cultivate your peak performance level over and again.

10) **Journaling:** Journaling is one of the most followed morning rituals by several successful people. They spend time writing every day to clear and calm their mind. Journaling has various proven benefits for a happier and productive day ahead.

Spend 15 minutes as your morning routine for journaling and writing whatever comes to your mind. Write things that you are grateful for, write your empowering affirmations, re-write your bigger goals, write your goals that you want to achieve today, write your priorities for the day, write down your thoughts and ideas, you can also dump your worries and write on how can you let go of the painful emotions and situations. Journaling is very powerful.

11) **Meditation:** A surest way to stay calm!

Meditation has been scientifically proven to be very effective in improving focus and creativity, decrease stress and anxiety, and changing the structure of our brain. Some people do meditate for hours while others just take a few minutes out of their morning routine. Meditation is one of the highly recommended and most common activities in the morning routine for all the highly successful people.

If you want to stay calm and stress-free for the entire day, start first with 5-7 minutes of meditation in your morning routine and increase this to 15-20 minutes if you continue to enjoy and see the benefits. It's quite natural that you may not be able to have the desired focus on meditation in your first few attempts, just focus on your breathing and gradually you will find yourself focused after a few days of continuity.

12) **Reading/podcast:** Incorporate reading in your morning routine because 'readers are leaders'. Reading is one of the simple and most effective parts of the morning routine for most successful people on this planet. Setting aside 10 minutes or more for reading a non-fiction book or listening to podcast or online course equips you to feed your mind with high quality-inputs and learnings that are required for your personal growth. The best way is to commit to a chapter on daily basis but if time doesn't permit, spend at least 10 minutes; get new ideas, breakthroughs and stay motivated for the rest of your day with the new learnings.

13) **Bond with loved ones:** Having a work-life balance is the key to success and perform at peak. Spending quality time with your loved ones early in the morning makes you feel positive and gives you a good enough reason to go out and give your best at work.

Showing your love and affection to your loved ones continue to strengthen your relationship with them and build trust. Not just that, cuddling them releases a lot of serotonin (Happy chemical-contributes to wellbeing and happiness) and that just boosts you up.

Pre-sleep Hour, another way to dominate!

There is no denial to the fact that morning rituals are very powerful. With the shift that morning rituals bring in life, so many people underestimate the power of evening or pre-sleep rituals but that's not the case with most successful people, with billionaires and with peak performers. They consistently adhere to pre-sleep rituals to evaluate their entire day, build relationships, and get the dose of positivity to set themselves up for the next day. And yes, they avoid screen-time (text messages and emails) during the pre-sleep hour. If you want to build your mental muscle for success these are some of the activities that you can incorporate in your pre-sleep rituals:

1) **Reflection:** Taking just a few minutes at the end of the day to reflect on and celebrate your wins gives you encouragement for the next day. It helps you overcome the discouragement that often comes with setbacks. Ask these powerful questions at the end of the day:

    a. 3 good things I have done today?

    b. Did I complete all my planned activities?

    c. What inspired me today?

    d. What should I focus on tomorrow?

    e. How can I do even better tomorrow?

2) **Journaling:** Journaling is as important in the pre-sleep hour as it is in the power-hour during the morning. Journal about:

    a. 3 things that I am grateful for today?

    b. Write 3 empowering affirmations.

    c. Write 3 empowering goals.

    d. 3 learnings today.

    e. Plan for tomorrow.

3) **Dose of positivity:** Bill Gates reads every night before diving in bed. What about you? Have a little downtime before you go to bed and read something positive and motivating books/text to continue to ignite you to unleash your potential. As mentioned earlier, "Leaders are readers". If you can spare some more time in your pre-sleep rituals, incorporate meditation to make you feel relaxed.

4) **Don't forget to spend quality time with your family.** Strengthening relationship with your loved ones is critical, schedule dedicated time in your evening schedule for your family, play with your kids and give personal attention to your spouse and parents to make them feel very special. You will be amazed to see the magic of these contributions towards your success.

Time to take Action:

All these rituals are backed by science and have a proven track record for various successful people. All you have to do is have them in your daily routine, consistently follow them during your 'power hour' 'Pre-sleep hour' and you will be able to witness your transformation to a different level. If you find it hard to have all of them in your routine, start with some of them and gradually incorporate the rest of them in your routine.

There are days when life intervenes and you have emergencies to deal with, how about your morning rituals on these days? Well, if you can't perform all the rituals, doing as much as you can in the morning is good or doing these later during the day is absolutely fine as well! But if not, no worries if it's just an occasional day or two as long you follow them more frequently.

All you have to consider is that the path of transformation initially looks harder but the benefits that you are going to reap afterward makes complete sense to do it anyway to be an extraordinary performer. Successful people also don't want to get up early but they do it anyway, extra-ordinary performers also don't want to sweat too hard but they do it anyway, being genius requires a little extra effort, little extra courage and little extra something that rest of the world doesn't do. So, do you want to be a genius? Do you want to be an extra-ordinary performer? Do you want to master the art of peak performance?

If Yes, Do it anyway! Set yourself up for the 'Power-hour' now!

"You'll never change your life until you change something you do daily. The secret of your success is found in your daily routine."

- John C. Maxwell

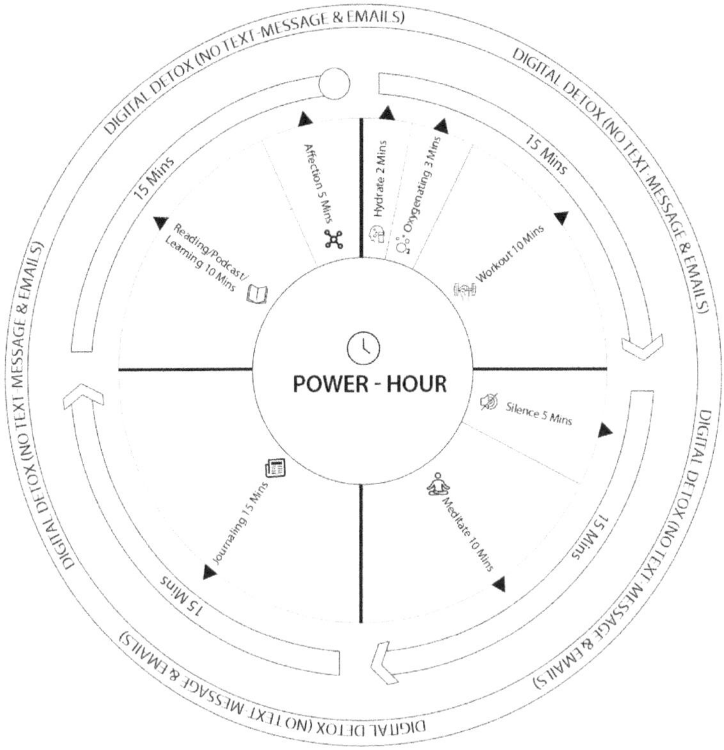

Recommended template for 'power-hour' rituals

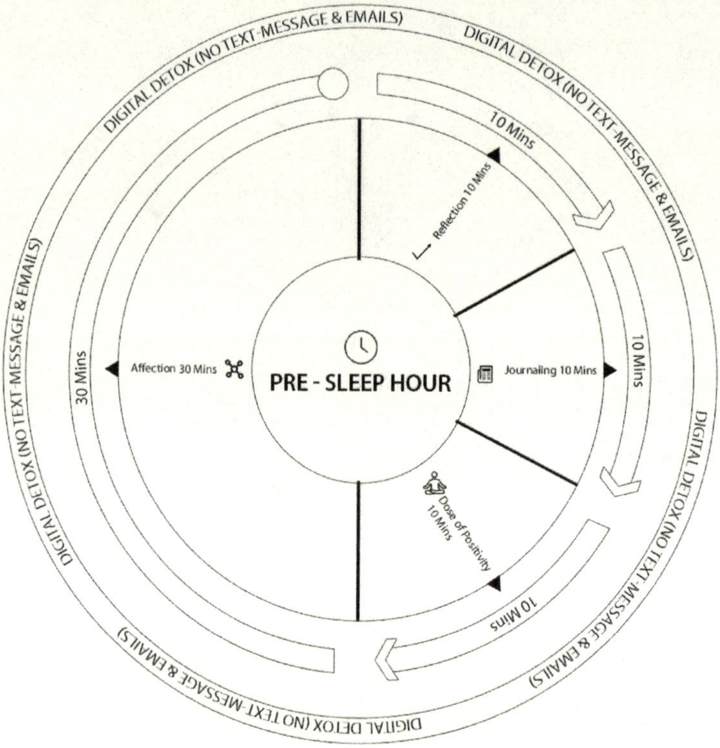

Recommended template for Pre-sleep hour

Chapter 15

TOOLS FOR EFFECTIVE COMMUNICATION

"Your ability to communicate determines how successful you're going to be in your life."

Effective communication is one of the key ingredients for any relationship whether it's at work or outside work. In any relationship, if you are able to communicate effectively, you can certainly see yourself doing so well in that particular area. Communication plays a gigantic role in our success.

So often, we feel it's quite simple but it's actually not. Now the question is what 'effective communication' is? For me, effective communication is, when the person/s you are communicating with understand the point you are trying to make, the way you want them to understand it. If their interpretation is in line with what you want them to understand then you have all the reasons to assume that you have communicated effectively.

Effective communication is power. There are a number of successful people who have mastered the art of communication and through this art, they have changed the world. How effective are your communication skills? Observe the relationships that affect you and your loved ones. How is your communication with them?

7-38-55 rule of communication.

"60% of all human communication is nonverbal body language; 30% is your tone, so that means 90% of what you're saying is not coming out of your mouth."

- Alex "Hitch" Hitchens

In the 1970s, Prof. Albert Mehrabian of UCLA, based on his research, claimed that the intent of any speaker is conveyed 7% through words, 38% through tone of voice and 55% through physiology (Body language). This rule is mostly taught in all the business workshops and events to emphasize on the importance of non-verbal elements in communication.

If we go by this rule, emails are only 7% effective, phone communication is 45% effective (7+38), and face to face communication is 100% (7+38 +55) effective. How true is this? Most of the business communication is being done through emails, and some of it through voice calls. So, it's hard to determine the proportion of this model in real sense. However, there is no way emails, voice and video calls can have the same impact as personal interaction.

The proportion of Mehrabian various elements has been questioned and not been proved except for certain specific and limited situations, but there is no denying that these 3 elements are present in all communication made in person, though the given proportion does not apply to all the communication in general. What is important to note here is 7-38-55 rule by Mehrabian explains the weight a listener gives on various elements of communication when a speaker is talking only about their feeling and attitude but it doesn't apply to all communications. Words carefully chosen and delivered, are powerful, but non-verbal elements (Tone of voice and physiology) play an even more significant role in overall communication. In order to make our words impactful, our tone of voice and body language has to be in congruence with the words that we speak.

NLP way for excellence in communication:

NLP, one of the powerful modern tools for personal excellence, it provides a number of tools and techniques to improve communication. In NLP, rapport is fundamental to all communications (which we are going to cover in this chapter). Then there is another concept called Sensory acuity which is the prerequisite for rapport and we will briefly cover it before moving onto rapport.

Sensory Acuity:

Sensory acuity is using our 5 senses to watch, listen and feel (in some cases) the subtle non-verbal signals that people are automatically sending so we can gain an understanding of how they are feeling and responding at any moment. This awareness can help us communicate even more effectively with them.

In short, Sensory acuity helps you gain an understanding of how someone is feeling at any moment and helps you choose what and how to communicate.

Think about how effectively you can influence your customer if you are a salesperson and have an awareness of their sensory acuity. How effectively you can influence your staff members if you are a manager and have awareness of their sensory acuity. How effectively you can influence your students if you are a teacher and have awareness of their sensory acuity.

How to use Sensory acuity:

Most of us already use sensory acuity automatically in our day-to-day life. Don't you use your senses to identify whether your spouse, boss, colleagues and friends are in good or bad mood simply by looking at them as soon as they walk into the room or the way they greet you first time by saying 'Hi' or 'Hello'? How you do that?

One of the simplest ways to do this is by comparing how they appear now versus how they normally do, or by recognizing certain non-verbal signals that the person is currently exhibiting and comparing these behaviors with our earlier interactions with them.

Some of the non-verbal interaction that we pay attention to is voice tonality, eye-focus, breathing-pattern (fast/slow, chest or abdomen), gestures (hand movement, body posture, etc.)

We can even use these signals with people whom we don't know or meeting with them for the first time. For example, if we are meeting our customer for the first time and during our casual chat before the meeting starts, if we pay attention to non-verbal signals when they talk about, frustration about current politics, infrastructure or any other experience that made them feel in a particular way then we get the understanding of how they feel at that moment and accordingly choose what and how to communicate with them. Isn't it magical?

Look for Pattern:

While there may be certain signs that strongly indicate how someone is feeling but not all the people use their body language in the same way, some people are more demonstrative than others, for example, somebody may reflect different signals while they are excited whereas another person may just be neutral. How to use our senses for situations like such? While reading their body language look for the pattern as people demonstrate the same response in more than one situation. For example, if someone folds his arm and display his angry behavior, be wary of him when he folds his arms next time. :)

While sensory acuity alone would rarely be sufficient in all the situations to identify how somebody is feeling but using our sensory acuity is quite useful to indicate when it might be useful to probe for more information.

These skills can be used in Interviews, sales meetings, appraisals meeting and are the foundation to build rapport which we are going to cover next and one of the most important elements of communication.

Rapport:

Poet, singer and civil rights activist Maya Angelou quoted;

"I've learned that people will forget what you said people will forget what you did but people will never forget how you made them feel"

- Maya Angelou.

Think about when you meet somebody, do you remember what they said or did or the feeling that is unforgettable? In most of the situations, what we feel becomes our unforgettable experience. Rapport helps the other person to feel better in a way appropriate to his or her situation. It helps the other person feel understood, connected and appreciated which is going to last longer than what you say and do for them

Rapport is an emotional connection with others wherein

both parties feel in sync. It helps in building a sense of comfort, responsiveness and confidence with someone. When you are in rapport with someone you enter into the other person's world and establish trust which is one of the key pre-requisite to have a good relationship with someone.

When you are in rapport with someone, you both have an emotional connection and understanding. You also respond very well to the body language of the other person, and want to be with the other person whether you are at work or in any other relationship.

How building Rapport helps in effective communication and performing at peak:

Building rapport is one of the key components of having effective communication which in turn helps to perform with excellence. Rapport is an ultimate tool for producing results at work. Being in rapport with colleagues at work works like magic. Rapport techniques are widely used in interviews, sales meetings, employee motivation and day-to-day working with colleagues in various corporates.

People usually have the tendency to work with people whom they like and trust. Rapport can help build likability and trustworthiness. Think of a time when you were completely in sync with others at work. What made you in sync with them? Chances are that there may be some commonality in the thinking patterns, beliefs, likes-dislikes, and background, etc., which made both of you understand and like each other. When you learn personal things about your colleagues and their likes-dislikes, you tend to find a common interest, it's nothing but rapport-building. Let's say you meet your colleagues on Monday and ask them how was their weekend and what they did. When they tell you they have been to a movie with family and if you have also been for the same movie then you start talking more about the same movie and are completely in sync.

How to build rapport at work:

Establishing rapport is one of the most important skills a person can have. When you are in rapport with your colleagues at work, you are more effective than otherwise, you can connect and understand your teams much faster, inspire them to perform at their best and produce the quality output. No matter what you want to achieve in your life whether it's earning millions, running successful teams and organization or anything, there is someone else who can help you be there, someone who knows how to effectively reach there faster. The way to have someone help you be there is to be in rapport with them, which creates the bond and a relationship of responsiveness.

Here are a few very effective techniques to build rapport:

1) Matching and Mirroring:

We all know, people tend to like people who are like themselves. I am always in sync with people who are like me and the same is the case with most of us. The key to be in an instant rapport with someone is to be like them and the quickest way to do is to match and mirror their physiology, tonality and words. Once we match and mirror someone unconsciously during our conversation, they start feeling that we are like them and it immediately builds trust and responsiveness.

Matching & mirroring physiology:

If we go by the 7-38-55 rule, Physiology, which is outside of our conscious awareness, plays a significant role (55%) ineffective communication. Thus, by mirroring and matching the physiology of the person we are communicating with, we can make ourselves like them and establish rapport with them easily. Each person uses different physiology. Matching and mirroring gestures, postures, energy level and body movements are quite effective and make the other person feel in sync with us. What is important to understand here is matching and mirroring should feel like happening unconsciously else it won't be impactful, also you don't have to give up who you are. You can still be in your own self and just match their physiology.

Matching Tonality:

Matching someone's tonality is key to make them feel you are like them, whether you are on a phone or conversing in person, match them vocally. Observe their pitch; is it high or low? Are they speaking fast or slow? Is the volume loud or quiet? Match their tonality and you will soon be finding yourself in rapport with them.

For example, if a person is speaking slow and in a low pitch then you would speak slow and in a low pitch to match with them and establish rapport. On the other hand if the person you are communicating with is speaking at a high speed and you are speaking very slowly then unconsciously you will not be in sync with them. Scientific studies have repeated this over and over again. When we can match someone vocally, we can start to get on the same page.

While matching the tonality, the copy-cat approach is not recommended at all. It should look like an unconscious matching.

Matching Keywords:

Matching the keywords used by another person is very useful in building rapport and it works like magic if you use the same tonality to those keywords. The words we use while conversing with others may have the same meaning but if those are not matching then it may not help to build rapport. For Example; if you are talking someone for the first time while watching cricket match and he says, "Virat Kohli is really energetic" and you match his keyword and say "Yes, he's really energetic" this matching of word help you establishing the rapport because the other person feels you are like him. What if you say? "His liveliness is amazing", it may have the same meaning but the person may not find himself in as much in sync as he was finding while you matched with his word 'energetic'. With conscious awareness matching, the keywords should be a natural part of communication as it increases our chances further for being in rapport with the ones we are conversing.

2) Commonality:

Commonality is one of the easiest and quickest way to build rapport with others. Find commonality between you and your colleagues at work, indulge in a healthy discussion that you both are passionate and interested about, and share your experience about that commonality. Finding some common ground will make you feel like you are in complete sync and you no longer have to establish barriers between you and the person you are conversing with. This sync and connect will help you make your relationship better with that persona whether it's at work or outside work.

3) Undivided attention:

Are you paying full attention while you are in conversation with someone?

In the current technological era of gazettes, we constantly switch around between our cell phones, laptops tablets and live conversations. We are not paying undivided attention to the people we are conversing with. While we feel we are doing multi-tasking at the same time but having our divided attention quickly sabotages any rapport that we have already established with our colleagues at work.

It's strongly recommended to be a good listener and pay undivided attention, especially when you are dealing with a human being. Stop replying to emails, text messages or answering any phone calls while you are in a conversation with someone. By doing this, you build a strong relationship and solid rapport with them at work.

4) WIIFM technique:

WIIFM is 'What's In It For Me?' WIIFM focuses on what benefits you can bring to the person you are communicating with? It is one of the most important techniques to build immediate rapport during sales meetings and interviews. While you are in a sales meeting, your prospect doesn't care about your product and the fact that you have to close the sale. What he cares about is what benefit this can bring for him and once he finds those benefits he will quickly be in sync with you and be in rapport. The same applies to interviews as well, while you are in an interview, it doesn't matter how qualified and intelligent you are unless you prove the interviewer how you can benefit the company. Once you establish the WIIFM relationship, you will quickly be in sync with the ones you care communicating with and can generate a much better outcome.

5) Water cooler Chatts:

Water cooler Chatts are the conversation that happens at work when colleagues take a short break during office hours. These Chatts helps employees to engage with others and have a healthy talk about their hobbies, interest and any other topic. While some of the managers do oppose as they feel these chatts as downtime but studies have proven that it helps employees build a relationship and build rapport amongst themselves. People not just feel open up with these Chatts but also get in sync and that helps them collaborate better for their work assignments. Therefore, ask thoughtful questions to the ones you are communicating with. This will allow them to open and share insights and build a connection with you. When you ask them a personal question, they get a feeling of you being concerned about their personal life which builds trust.

Are you participating in healthy water cooler talks? If not, participate and get involved and ask thoughtful questions, these informal conversations will certainly help you build relationship with your colleagues, and the connection that you have established with these talks helps you do wonders with your work relationship.

To summarize, rapport building is very important for effective communication and all these techniques show we can build rapport with anyone and create an environment of trust and responsiveness which helps in effective communication.

Exercise:

1) Are you in sync with people at work?
2) Try and build rapport with your colleagues at work and see how it impacts your communication with them?

Chapter 16

FALL IN LOVE WITH F.E.A.R (FOCUS. ENERGY. ADAPTABILITY. RESILIENCE.)

F-Focus:

"Your Inability to focus is the death of your productivity."

Focus is nothing but how attentive we are to anything that we do. Our ability to focus determines our level of performance. Staying focussed is one of the key pre-requisites to boost our performance in any area of our life. All the successful people and peak performers have mastered the art of focus and it has helped them accomplish the level of success that they wished for. Staying focused is not difficult but it requires taking some actions, developing the habits and implementing strategies to enhance productivity.

Do you often find yourself losing focus when working on tasks? It is not unusual to find ourselves losing focus, especially in today's world where there are too many things that can distract us. Like stumbling over to the phone, getting lost in the notifications of social media, stopping by the desk of a colleague to chit chat, addiction to mobile games, mental and physical clutter that makes you unsystematic and disorganized. These little things make a dramatic difference in our ability to focus, and hinder your potential to perform at our best.

Are there too many tasks and deadlines and not enough days? The workload creeps up on you slowly and then all at once. So, how do you manage to accomplish these everyday tasks without letting outside distractions and stressors get in the way? Fortunately, there are various techniques available that might help you remain focused.

Here are a few quick hacks to develop a laser-like focus and excel your performance:

1) Schedule around your energy:

Schedule your most important task (MIT) in your most energetic time slot during your workday. Researches show we have more mental energy in the morning hours, it's the prime time, so schedule your prime task during your prime-time slot and stay away from distraction during that time. Stay in the tight bubble of total focus, no water-cooler talks, no social media, no roaming around the office and no distraction at all while you are performing your most important tasks in your most energetic time.

2) Pomodoro technique or 25/5 Rule

It's one of the proven time management philosophies that helps the user to stay focus, stay fresh and avoid mental fatigue. Under this technique, you break your workday into 25-minute chunks separated by five-minute of short breaks. You have to complete each work in 25 minutes and take a 5-minute break. Since you know you have to complete the work in 25 minutes, so you stay focus and your short break after every 25 minutes will help you avoid mental fatigue.

Applying this technique initially may not bring positive results but if used correctly for a reasonable time, it can be very helpful.

There are several researches that say you can't stay focussed for longer than 25-30 minutes. However, if you feel 25/5 rule has to be changed statistically then you can modify this to make it work for you but the idea is to work in cycles and have short breaks after each interval to stay focus.

3) Focus on Friendly Diet:

The supply of focus on a friendly diet that has nutrients and healthy fats can have a huge impact on focus for an extended period. Certain foods have nutrition punch to boost your productivity and focus. Drinking more water (to stay hydrated and energetic), blueberries (they are loaded with nutrients and antioxidants that help in stay productive), avocados (they are low in sugar, high in protein that helps you in sustain focus), leafy-green vegetables (helps our neurons communicate better and fire more efficiency).

At the same time, certain foods like Sugar, Alcohol, Muffins, heavily processed carbs and fruit juices with high sugar, etc. can lead to lowering our energy and focus.

4) Email and social media rituals to minimize distractions:

Robin Sharma, rightly said, "Addiction to distraction is the death of your creative production." Our addiction to social medial and emails has been the killer for our productivity and focus in most of the cases.

How can you stay focus on your work if your phone keeps buzzing with Instagram notifications and your laptop keeps notifying you about your Facebook feed? Set some rituals and stay away from such distractions. While you may feel it only takes a few mins to quickly go through these updates but that's a serious killer of your focus.

While we understand checking email is mandatory if it falls in your work nature but even if it's mandatory there have to be some rituals for checking those at specific time-intervals so you are not distracted when you are engaged in most important tasks.

Set your emails and social media rituals to multiply your productivity and focus. Keeping your phone on airplane mode or social media notifications off during your workday is strictly recommended to stay focus.

5) Meditation and Exercise:

"Anything that is good for your heart is good for your brain."

Exercise can make our blood moving throughout our body and it can make the grey part of our brain grow which helps in learning and memorizing. There are plenty of researches showing regular exercise improves attention span. Spending 15-30 minutes of physical exercise is strongly recommended to have better concentration.

Meditation is the surest way to build focus. Sitting with closed eyes and observing your breath helps you stay focused and keeps you calm and stress-free. Start with 5 minutes of meditation and gradually increase the duration if you continue to find it beneficial.

6) Set daily goals:

Having a long term goal is great but focusing on the 10-year goal is not easy. Setting small daily goals will wire our brain for success and when it's linked with the reward mechanism, getting rewarded for accomplishing daily goals will continue to motivate for tomorrow's goal.

E- Energy: Stay energetic to perform at peak:

Are you feeling devoid of energy and enthusiasm? Are you finding yourself totally knocked out? Alas! Low energy means low productivity and no optimal performance.

But as the popular phrase goes 'Life belongs to the energetic', always remember, no time management system or productivity application can ever substitute the requirement for high energy. This, in turn, ensures peak performance and optimal results in all your endeavors. Your energy levels are directly proportional to your productivity, which means higher the energy levels, higher is the performance level leading to higher productivity.

Feeling energetic is the key to getting what you want to be accomplished in life. Studies show that you are more likely to feel good about yourself when you feel energetic. On the other hand, when you feel exhausted, things that you generally enjoy doing like decorating your living room might seem like a task which can make you feel overwhelmed and stressed.

So if you are working on something or attempting to achieve something but are feeling that the results are somehow not optimal, stop and analyze if you are feeling adequately energetic and if not, work on boosting your energy levels first so as to reach your peak-performance.

How to stay energetic?

Some of the quick hacks to boost the energy are to sleep properly, eat the right type of food, exercise on a regular basis, take regular breaks after every 25-45 minutes of work and stay stress-free. Focus on what makes you happy and always surround yourself with positive thoughts, emotions, and people. They will not only lift you but also motivate you to reach the zenith of your performance and touch great heights.

A-Adaptability

"All failure is failure to adapt, all success is successful adaptation."

- Max McKeown

How adaptable you are? Oh! Sorry, let me first explain what adaptability is? Your Adaptability refers to how easily you can adapt to any change. It entails how open you are to new ideas, new concepts, changed situations and being able to work as the situation demands. The more adaptable and flexible you are, the more are the chances for you to perform at your best and be successful. Now tell me how adaptable you are?

If you are puzzled why adaptability is important then let me help you understand that adaptability is one of the critical success factors for all the peak performers. In today's fast-paced world, life adaptability is a sought-after skill. Those who are adaptable are least bothered by unfavorable situations and they know better ways of coping with them. With this adaptability, they change the strategy rather than avoiding the task. They powerfully influence the way they handle mistakes and failures and accomplish their goals in various areas of their life.

How adaptable are you?

How adaptable you are to new processes, new policies, and new technology at your workplace? Are you enthusiastically responding to the changes? Adaptability is little more than being flexible. It is about being adaptable to things, even outside of our comfort zone. Adaptability is not something that you are born with, it has to be developed with regular practice.

Quick hacks to be adaptable:

1) Primary Motivation:

To adapt to any change or any situation, your primary motivation plays an important role. When you feel adaptable to the changes, it can bring long term gains then you are motivated to take short term pains. For example, if relationship is your key driver then think about how beautiful your relation will be with others after you adapt.

2) Mental Preparation:

To adapt to unpredictable opportunities of the moment, mental preparation plays the key part. A mindset that is open and has the willingness to accept the changes can adapt very fast.

3) Comfort zone to Stretch Zone:

Nothing great can be achieved by staying in comfort zone. Most of the growth happens when we stretch ourselves beyond our comfort zone. Stretch zone is the best place to be in and most of the peak performers stay in this zone. Moving ourselves from comfort zone to stretch zone will improve our ability to be adaptable but we need to make sure that while moving from comfort zone to stretch we don't move too far to reach a 'panic zone' as this is not the best place to be in.

4) Accept changes:

By nature, we are programmed to resist changes. Start accepting the small-small changes and gradually your muscles will be reprogrammed to accept changes which can be a good starting point to be conditioned to adapt to bigger changes when it comes your way.

Adaptability is one of the important qualities to cope up with fast-paced changes that modern lifestyle demands. By applying these simple hacks we can improve our ability to adapt ourselves as per the demand of the situation. Ultimately, this helps us in enhancing our performance in various areas of our life.

R-Resilience:

Do you know, why some people thrive in the face of challenge and adversity at work, while others panic and suffer? Why some people recover from setbacks and challenges whereas others get stuck into those?

Those who have adopted the process of being resilient are the ones who are able to thrive on the face of setback, challenges and stress. They stand tall like a strong tree and are able to handle the storm whereas others aren't. Resilience is how we bounce-back despite any adverse circumstances. What about you? How are you responding to the tough times at work and in any area of your life? Are you resilient or not?

How resilience helps in excelling performance:

Resilience is not a trait that people either have it or not. It involves how you are responding to the situation, which thoughts and behavior you are producing and what actions you are taking. Resilience is not a passive quality but an active process on how we take and handle various situations of our life. Being resilient increases our ability to perform under pressure and to stay stress-free despite adverse circumstances.

"The human capacity for burden is like bamboo- far more flexible than you'd ever believe at first glance."

-Jodi Picoult

We need to be resilient, we need to bounce back with fervor, only then we can maximize our performance levels and reach our peak performance. Resilience makes one capable of staying calm in times of adversity and one continues paving the way towards prosperity and success thereby enhancing one's performance efficiency. When it comes to professional world and stringent workplace settings, we all know how one has to deal with quite a lot of problems ranging from immense work pressure, discrimination issues, lack of effective leadership or motivation, unfair wages/ inappropriate appraisals or bullying colleagues. This is where one's capacity to bear and bounce back comes into action. This is what can empower one to touch the zenith of one's performance capacity.

7 C's to stay Resilient:

There are several little things one should keep in mind to build resilience. Here are the 7 "C"s guidelines to be resilient which are as follows:

Competence: Building competency is the key to give you the feeling of knowing and this strong feeling makes you competent to handle specific situations in various areas of life.

Confidence: Focus on your strengths and the best in you to stay confident. Believe in your abilities, remember and recall your accomplishments to give you the dose confidence to bounce-back.

Connection: Have a good social connection. Several researches show that the primary factors in resilience are about caring and having supportive relationships within and outside the family. Relationships that create love and trust and offer encouragement and reassurance help bolster a person's resilience.

Coping: Learn on how to effectively cope up with various adverse and challenging situations of day-to-day life.

Control: Don't try to control the uncontrollable, there are certain things that you can control but certain things you can't. We can't have control on the outside situation but we can control the inside, be strong when there is a tough time and bounce back.

Character: Have a solid set of character with strong moral values to identify the good in bad to feel positive. Happy people don't have a perfect life, they make the best of what they have rather than having the best of everything. Find out what's good about that adverse situation? How it can benefit you?

Continue your journey: Challenges and setbacks are a part of life and sometimes challenges teach what success can't. Accept challenges that come your way, it's not the end of your life, Inhale-Exhale, move on and come back even stronger.

"You may have to fight a battle more than once to win it."

- Margaret Thatcher

Chapter 17

WHAT MAKES GREAT PEOPLE GREAT?

"Don't practice until you get it right, practice until you can't get it wrong."

Practice

Have you ever heard 'Practice makes a man perfect'? I am sure you have. We all know if we like to master any skill then we have to practice, practice and practice. Learning any skills needs repetition, as you continue to repeat your tend to get better day-by-day.

Now the question is, is it just practice (repetition) that makes us perfect? When we talk about Practice, it's the quantity that we are talking about. Accordingly, the more we repeat any activity, the better we will become in that particular skill.

Can we shoot for 8 hours without any technique and become perfect just by practice? Can we study for 8-10 hours on any subject every day for 3 years and be perfect in that just by practice? Can a Cricketer practice for 6 hours every day without any strategy and be perfect?

What's your answer to these questions? I am sure you must be trying to brainstorm and after some brainstorming, you might be thinking it's not just 'Practice', there has to be something else that is required apart from practicing, that helps us 'master' or be 'Perfect' in particular skills or subject. But, what's that? Practice has to be 'perfect' to help us to be a perfectionist in that skill. It has to be 'Perfect Practice', not just practice.

What is perfect practice then?

When we talk about Perfect Practice, we refer to the quality of the practice than quantity, Perfect practice has to be a strategic, purposeful and consistent way to improve. We may call it an 'Intelligent Practice' 'Perfect Practice' or 'Purposeful Practice'. When we follow the elements of perfect practice, the probability of mastering the skills and performing with excellence is much higher.

To summarize, Perfect Practice requires a focused goal and conscious plan for improvement. It is one of the Golden rules to master any skill, achieve excellence, be a perfectionist and Perform at your peak.

Perfect Practice

"You can shoot 8 hours a day, but if your technique is wrong, all you become is good at shooting the wrong way. Get the fundamental down and the level of everything you do will rise."

- Michael Jordan (NBA Legend)

"Practice does not make perfect. Only perfect practice makes perfect."

- Vince Lombardi

You can study for as many hours as you want but in order to master that subject you have to read the right content, with right planning, right strategy with focused goal to reach excellence and be a perfectionist.

Let's say as a Student, you see how other students are getting good grades, you are learning their strategies, watching various videos of successful students, but if you can't take action and grow around what you have learned, you can you be a successful student. Well, you can't.

So let's start taking action, you may make some mistakes in the beginning but that's a part of the process. That's how you will keep learning and modifying your practice strategies and by formulating the 'Perfect' one is what will make you successful.

To cut it short, only perfect Practice makes you perfect. The key to perfection is to strive for excellence.

Perfect means, "Free from all flows and never mess up."

Excellence means, "Doing the work in the best possible way, to the best of your ability and available information."

As a human being, we tend to make some mistakes initially but the more we practice and identify where we are going wrong and correcting them continuously, we gradually move towards good to better and to excellence eventually. So our effort should be to strive for excellence. So, are you ready to strive for excellence? Here are 4 key habits that you can adopt to tread to excellence: Identifying Core Skills, Practice what matters most, get Feedback and never stop Practicing.

Deliberate practice:

After learning what Practice and Perfect Practice is, there is another important concept called 'Deliberate Practice' (described by Anders Ericsson, Florida State Psychology professor in one of his famous book 'PEAK') is the process of working in a specific, purposeful and strategic way to improve any skill.

The concept of 'Deliberate practice applies to pretty much anything that we can imagine and has been used by everyone ranging from best musicians to Olympic winners to become the best at their skill.

What's deliberate practice? And how using this can help us get better and parade from good to best? To understand this further, we will quickly understand how Anders Ericsson has shared the concept of deliberate practice in his book: Deliberate practice refers to a special type of practice that is purposeful and systematic. While regular practice might include mindless repetitions, deliberate practice requires focused attention and is conducted with the specific goal of improving performance.

To understand this, let's first understand how we learn and improve any skill?

Think about how you learnt driving a car, as a beginner, everything is new and scary and our brain is naturally attentive to every detail as we work hard to understand the basics.

However, as we progress—either from getting lessons from a friend or coach or maybe watching a tutorial video—we get past that first scary part. Now, we are good enough to go through the motions, doing the basic moves over and over until they become automatic.

Eventually, we hit a point where our skills are "good enough". We can do the thing we set out to do. And that's where our improvement plateaus.

At this point, no more practice of going through the motions will make us not improve. And to most people, it's acceptable. But if you want to become a master or an expert, you need to break out of this phase.

Good enough is not enough

Various researches have shown that once a person reaches a 'good-enough' or 'Satisfactory-level', the additional years of practice don't lead to any improvement. This is the reason, Doctor who have been practicing for more than 25 years may not be better than the one with only 3-5 years of experience who is continuously putting his efforts in improving. Automated skills deteriorate in the absence of deliberate efforts.

So, let's not be satisfied with this level of performance and continue to learn effective tools and techniques on how you can improve your performance even further, If you are a writer, learn effective ways or you can be more creative and write fast. If you are an engineer, find out effective tools that can automate your manual efforts in a short span of time, If you are a runner, find out how you can complete the run in lesser time, to continue to improve your performance. Therefore, 'Deliberate practice' is highly recommended.

So what you should do once you reach an acceptable level and want to improve continuously? This is where deliberate practice makes sense.

The difference between "automatic" repetitive practice and the more purposeful "deliberate" practice comes down to **knowing where you need improvement and focusing intensely on getting better in that area.** Deliberate practice is taking a systematic and specific approach to improvement that builds over time, rather than simply doing the same thing over and over and over.

The key is, in knowing what areas need your attention, and that requires Feedback. And it's not just feedback, its constant Feedback and mentorship, which tells you what steps to take to get even better.

Deliberate practice is not a magic wand that will change the things for best overnight, it's all about working hard in a deliberate and purposeful manner.

Steps of Deliberate practice:

1) **Define measurable and effective goal:** Having a defined goal helps a lot in putting your best efforts. Define the general goal and break it to small measurable and achievable goals. With each of these small goals, take them one by one and continue to work on those with a realistic expectation of improvement.

Purposeful practice is all about putting a bunch of baby steps together to reach a long term goal. If your goal is to write a book, break it into several measurable and achievable goals, like writing 10 pages every week with the required quality of content, etc.

If your goal is to successfully crack any competition exam then you can break the entire course into various parts and come up with a date of completion for each part, continue with your efforts for each part and get better day-by-day.

2) **Focus:** Deliberate practice requires focus on the goal. The intensity with which the practice is to be performed should be at its peak. Deliberate practice doesn't need to set aside a major portion of your day practicing. In fact, most studies agree that the success of deliberate practice comes down to focus and intensity than to duration.

3) **Consistent Feedback Mechanism by mentors:** As mentioned earlier, consistent feedback by mentors or experts is one of the fundamental and key elements to make deliberate practice work. Feedback mechanism has to be the one that

gives us insights into each and every aspect of our progress and helps us in areas where fine-tuning is required. And this fine-tuning is required consistently to raise our performance bar every other time.

4) **Getting out of Comfort Zone:** This is one of the most important parts of purposeful practice. In order to perform extra-ordinary, we have to push beyond the accepted and comfortable level. Putting more efforts than what is easy is Must. This applies to almost all kinds of skills.

As mentioned earlier, if we want to achieve something that we have never achieved then we have to do something that we have never done before. There are several proven evidences to prove this. We have to challenge our abilities and increase our efforts gradually to improve our capabilities

If we never push ourselves beyond our comfort zone, we will never improve and there is no way we can perform at peak without improving on our skills in consistent manner.

What we have to be careful about is we have to push ourselves to a level which our mind and body can reasonably sustain. Pushing our limits gradually is the most ideal scenario to test our potential. Once the set level is attained we have to set a higher benchmark to push ourselves but if we can't attain those higher benchmarks then we have to continue the one we already attained for some more time. This will allow our mind and body to get used to it until it becomes a part of our comfort zone. Once it reaches the comfort zone then we can push it gradually and continue the process.

5) **Passion and Love:** Find out what you love and are passionate about. It's important to be interested in the skills that you want to expertise in. This plays a huge role in how quickly and effectively you can improve on your skills. The intensity of your efforts is entirely different if you do something you are passionate about. You will have an automated inner push to continue learning and practicing with focus for hours and hours even when you are practicing out of your comfort zone.

We all have an incredible ability to improve our skills, and deliberate practice in a focused environment is the mantra to maximize our potential as long as we put in the work. Anyone can improve, but it requires the right approach. If you are not performing well doesn't mean you are not talented; it's because you are not practicing the right way.

"Caliber of deliberate practice determines the quality of your performance."

Chapter 18

BE A DOER, KNOWING IS NOT ENOUGH!

I remember, once I was addressing a set of people and sharing some insights on a topic when someone within the audience said, "I already know this" and to my surprise few others also joined him saying they have already learned about the same topic earlier. Then my question was, "Why are you not acting on it? What stops you from implementing what you have already learned?" There was impenetrable silence! Ask yourself this question if you are also in the same situation, do you know something which is important and can do wonders but not putting the same into work.

In this digital era, we have access to a plethora of knowledge flow from all over the places. Knowledge is not the challenge, the actual challenge is to convert our knowledge into action. The internet era has made access to information with a lot of ease. We are overwhelmed with information via podcasts, TED Talks, Online articles, blogs, etc., and we are not shying away from learning anything that makes us aware, gives us insights, and enhances our knowledge base. However, when it comes to acting upon our knowledge, there is still a wide gap between what we know and what we employ in real life. We employ far less than what we know. Isn't it true for you?

We know the importance of exercising and healthy eating but we don't put this into practice.

We know how to reduce weight but we don't hit the gym or engage ourself in a workout session.

We know the importance of making goals and following daily routines but we never made one for us.

We know how to make our relationship better but we never apply those in our day-to-day life.

We know more about our skills than we actually use them.

Are you more of a learner or doer? I agree, In order to do something the first step is to know and we are doing okay when it comes to knowing or learning but if we evaluate our level of performance with a level of knowledge, we will find that we are under utilizing our knowledge in various areas of our life. Only a few of us are actually doers of what we know and most of us are not putting our knowledge into action. While we agree, there is always going to be some gap but the wider the gap is more we are under-utilizing our knowledge.

"Knowing is not enough we must apply, willing is not enough we must do."

-Johann Vann Goethe.

Disconnection between what you know in your head and what comes out of your hand is quite different and that is the gap we want to address. In order to address this, we have to first identify how wide the gap is? To what extent we fully perform what we know? What are the reasons for this gap? How to bridge the gap?

Reasons why we don't do what we know.

Impression of Action:

We often confuse ourselves with planning or talking equals to action but it's actually not. When we start planning on anything we assume the action has started and we feel we are putting our knowledge to action but that's a trick to make us believe that we are in action mode. What we have to make ourselves understand here is planning or talking before taking any action is important but these talks or planning are not action yet.

Dominant emotions of yours:

Fear is one of the most dominant emotions that hold us back from taking any action. It's so deeply rooted that it creates a lot of hesitation and due to this we know that we should take the action but still we keep waiting in the wings and most of us never take off. In most of the cases, we feel confident when we learn new things but when it comes to action, somewhere in the back of our mind, fear flame exaggerates that says "it's dangerous", "it's risky", "Avoid" and that widens the gap between what we know and what we do.

Fear can cripple in different forms; fear of failure, fear of the unknown, fear of unpredictable, fear of competition, etc.

I'm not perfect yet!

What people know they feel they are not perfect yet and they need to learn more to gain more knowledge so they learn more by buying books, attending workshops, listening more podcasts and taking more courses but that doesn't help and widens the gap further because the problem of 'not doing' still remains the same whereas the 'level of knowledge' keeps increasing.

Here, what we have to realize is, if we don't act on what we have already learned, we will get the same result as if we have not learned anything. Don't wait for perfection, go out take action, make mistakes and learn from those mistakes to continue to improve.

Personality traits;

Some of us are not action-oriented, whereas some of us give a number of excuses for not taking any action. Some of us think learning and knowing something is sufficient and they keep learning but they don't act upon this.

Why knowing is not sufficient:

Knowing will not bring the change, doing will!

Knowledge means nothing if you don't apply what you learned. Knowing something will not get you anything unless you act upon this. Ask yourself, why you have spent time acquiring the knowledge that you acquired.

There is no learning without doing:

The key here is that learning requires doing. The key point is that knowing is not really learning, knowing is just the first ingredient to start the process. When we start doing and reflecting on our doing then slowly new learning emerges.

How to bridge knowing-doing gap

Convert fear to feedback:

Fear and procrastination belong to the same family, when you are in fear, procrastination comes in between and holds you back to widen the knowing-doing gap. One of the strong presupposition of NLP says 'There is no failure, only feedback' if you try, there are chances for you to succeed but if you don't it does not mean that you have lost, rather take it as a learning. When you try for things and take action, this process itself gives a number of learning that you can't get without trying for those. And these learnings are certainly going to help you eventually.

Shift your paradigm:

Your paradigms are the ones allowing you to think in a certain way and act in a certain way. Therefore, unless you change the mental programming running in your subconscious mind, nothing is going to change. To shift your paradigm you have to constantly repeat the habit that you want to incorporate.

Walk your talk approach:

Making use of what you know requires action because action produces result, without action all the knowledge is useless.

Set a deadline:

Setting a deadline to do what you know helps you strop dragging this any further. When you set a deadline, you are training yourself to complete the action within the time limit and it's quite effective.

By implementing our knowledge in our day-to-day life, we will be able to have the real-time experience of knowledge and that experience will continue to give us the feedback to bring the change that we would like to see in our life. This change can be installing a new habit, implementing new skills at our work, trying new routines for better productivity, new behavior to improve the performance, etc.

Chapter 19

SKILL OR WILL

Skill Vs Will:

If somebody is not been able to perform as per the expected level, the first question that comes to the mind is, "Is it a lack of will or lack of skill?"

When the 'God of Cricket' said "Main khelega"....

In a cricket match between India Vs Pakistan in the year 1989: team India was in a tough situation. The young Sachin Tendulkar had come out to bat, Batsman Navjot Sidhu was already at the crease and four were already down for 38 runs. Since it was a green-top wicket and Waqar Younis was a super-fast bowler, team India was going through a very difficult time at the crease. Waqar Younis came to bowl and slammed the ball in the middle of the wicket. The ball hit squarely on Tendulkar's nose. He fell down and was bleeding profusely. Physio ran towards him for help, Navjot Sindhu also ran for his rescue. When everybody was waiting for Sachin to be carried on a stretcher, he spoke those 2 words, he said to Physio and Sidhu that he won't go out for treatment. He said, "Main Khelega" which means I WILL PLAY.

When he said those words it was his 'will' that made him stand up and play at that time inspite of his bleeding nose. We all know the heights he reached in his life with the combination of his skills and will.

What are Skills?

Skills refer to the knowledge and capability of any person to perform any task. Every task requires a different level of skill.

Skill plays a significant role in how an individual performs. A person may have very good skills in performing one task whereas he may not have very good skills in performing any other task.

What is Will?

It is an individual's desire to complete a particular task, based on motivation, incentive, attitude, and personal feeling about that particular task. It is what we are willing to do to achieve our goals or to do our job as required and to really perform above the level what is required. In the case of Sachin Tendulkar, his skills didn't come for his rescue in the earlier example. It was his will that made him stand tall and face the music.

In order to have somebody perform at peak, having both skill-will at the highest level is like 'Hip-Hip-Hurrah'. A person may have all the required skills, knowledge and experience to perform but it is of no use if he is not willing to execute his plans.

Your 'will' must be Stronger than the 'Skill'

- Mohammed Ali

Skill-will matrix:

It is used to assess an individual's skill level and willingness to perform any task. Several leaders prefer to follow the skills-will quadrant to decide on what type of individuals they would like to have in their teams and accordingly;

High will and High skill: Preferable.

If you are in this category, you are very close to performing to the best of your capability if you continue to focus with the required energy and take necessary actions at the right time.

High Will and Low skill: Can be considered.

If fall under this, you have to work on sharpening your skills so you can perform better than what you have been doing so far.

Low will and High skill: Put on hold.

If you come under this category, you need to work on your motivation. Be confident about your skills and stay enthusiastic to take the necessary action. Also remember, your talent has no value unless you develop the will power and execute.

Low will and low skills: To be rejected.

This is a very tricky combination to get the best of you. You don't just have to work on your motivation but also have to sharpen your skills to stay productive. The path to peak performance seems difficult and requires a lot of effort on both skill-will perspective, but yes, it's possible.

Chapter 20

11 MAXIMS TO PERFORM AT PEAK

11 Maxims for peak performance:

"Maxims are the germs of all excellence."

Maxim #1. Own your life.

You are living in a world that is too busy to care about you and your core strengths, so the responsibility falls on you to apply your strengths every day. Take ownership for all areas of your life and see how you are performing in each of those areas. Never blame others, you are the captain of your own ship, take control and move on. Keep a mirror with you and look into it in the time of trouble. It'll show you the source of the problem and solution to your problems.

Ask yourself: Do I take 100% responsibility for all my successes and failures?

Maxim #2. Be coachable.

Even if you are at your best; have an open mind and be coachable. Who knows you get some clue that helps you to perform a fraction better. Listen to your mentors, observe people who are in the same field, learn from people having special skills.

Ask yourself: Am I open to learn and grow?

Maxim #3. Always a student.

Knowledge is the power, it opens your mind and unleashes your potential. With knowledge you have better choices, when you know more you do more. If you want to stay ahead and want to get better in doing what you do then keep learning new tricks, new technologies and new ways to master your craft. Be a lifelong learner and have an attitude of 'always a student' with a growth mindset. Have a dedicated time of 30 minutes or more in your daily schedule and sharpen your core skills. A willingness to learn and evolve is invaluable when it comes to attaining personal excellence and achieving peak performance.

Ask yourself: Do I have the 'always a student' attitude?

Maxim #4. You Vs you.

You are your toughest rival. Find out, are you better today than you were yesterday? Excellence in performance is all about self-improvement, keep raising your standards, aim to perform a fraction better than a day before. You can also use other great performers as extra inspiration for your improvement but your toughest competitor is you.

Ask yourself: Am I better today than what I was before?

Maxim #5. Ask empowering questions.

These 3 powerful questions can kindle fire in your belly. Ask yourself every single day:

Morning - How will I be a genius today? (Intention)

Evening- How was I genius today? Did I give my 100%? (Refection & Accountability)

Night- What needs to get better? (Accountability)

Maxim #6. Be authentic.

Here's the Chinese proverb that you can follow "Tension is who you think you should be. Relaxation is who you are."

You are at your best when you behave the way you are. When you copy somebody, it's not you and won't get the best out of you. Be with your natural instinct and bring your originality to play and you will perform at your peak. Be authentic and keep it real.

Ask yourself: Am I keeping it real?

Maxim #7. Complexity to simplicity.

Don't fall in love with complexity. Simplicity is what takes you where you want to be. Don't overthink, just focus on the basics. Just go out in the middle and enjoy doing what you are doing. Follow the KISS formula; Keep It Simple and Straightforward. Success comes with staying consistently on fundamentals.

Ask yourself: Am I following simplicity?

Maxim #8. Execution is the key.

No Ideas work unless you do the work. Having a great idea that can change the world won't make any impact unless that idea is being executed. Are you one of them getting a lot of ideas by reading books, going to workshops, attending seminars and thinking then why your life is not changing? Well, it will never change unless you execute your ideas. Your ideas in your mind won't get you anything unless you bring them to work. Talk less, do more is the mantra! Do it and be the genius for this world, for the country, for your community, for your loved ones and if you can't be genius for anybody, be a genius for yourself! Get this done for you!

Ask yourself: Am I taking action to be a genius?

Maxim #9. Celebrate small victories.

List out your top 5 targets that you wish to accomplish during the course of the day for you to feel the productive day. Go crazy for a few minutes and celebrate after you achieve each target. Do this consistently for a few months and you will see stunning results. These moments of victory will keep you pumped up and stay focused. Celebrating after every accomplishment will navigate you from negative bias to positive.

Ask yourself: Did I celebrate my victories today?

Maxim #10. Invest in yourself.

This is the best investment you can ever have that can get you 1000x returns in whatever areas you are in. Go learn new skills, new techniques, newer and quicker ways of doing what you do, learn productivity hacks and be a better person than what you are today. The amount spent on a new smartphone will get depreciated after few months but the amount invested in your personal and professional learning will get you exponential return for the rest of your life. The choice is yours!

Ask yourself- Am I investing in personal and professional upgradation?

Maxim #11. Be consistent.

Greatness lies in consistency. Excellence is not doing great things or giving your 100% one day, one week or one month, it's about continuing your masterpiece every single day.

Ask yourself- Am I consistently giving my best every single day?

Chapter 21

LAST BUT NOT THE LEAST, USE THESE 7 'POWER' AND BE A GENIUS!

#1. Power of 'Power'

The easiest way to feel you are powerless is to feel you have no power. Don't feel yourself powerless, your potential is nearly limitless. People who have grown from nowhere to the peak are no different than you, they have the same power as you have but they have made the choice of realizing their potential and acted on this consistently... You also have the power! Go from "Can I" to "I Can" and from "I am not good enough" to "I am good enough" and you will see the magic happening.

#2. Power of 'Shut up'

You have the power to live your life the way you want, you are the captain of the ship, you are the director of your movie and you can project any movie to this world that you want. Just say 'Shut up' to your inner voice if it holds you back, say 'Shut up' to each and every one who tells you, "you can't do it".

#3. Power of 'Yes'...

Figure out what are those opportunities to whom you said 'No' in the past but you are going to say 'Yes' today onwards. Say 'Yes' to exceptionalism. Say 'Yes' to the sharpening of your skills. Say 'Yes' to invest in your personal development. Say 'Yes' to get ready to change inside-out. Say 'Yes' to have a challenging goal and stay committed to that goal no matter what. Say 'Yes' to everything that you feel can bring positive changes in your life. The more you say 'Yes' to new and challenging opportunities, the better are the chances for you to unleash your potential.

#4. Power of 'No'

When you say 'Yes' to one goal that is your deepest desire and commit to focus on achieving it, you automatically get the power of saying 'No' that doesn't align with that goal. When you say 'Yes' to positivity, you get the power of saying 'No' to negativity. When you say 'Yes' to success, you get the power to say 'No' to your fears and excuses. Saying 'No' to what is not aligned is what takes you closer to who you want to be or what you wish for.

#5. Power of I'm....

The word you replace after "I am" has an incredible impact on your life because this is what you believe about yourself. If you say "I am Powerful", you think, act and behave like a powerful person but it's entirely opposite if you replace it with something powerless. The word that you put after "I'm" has to be empowering enough to make you believe that 'everything is possible' and 'you have all the qualities that are required to be a successful person'. Try to do it for 90 days followed by action and you will be amazed to see the difference this will make.

#6. Power of Choice:

Spend the day in bed, or get to work. Sit on the couch, or step out to work. Be a genius or continue to be what you are. You have dozens of choices to make every day. The power of choice is amazing, what you choose is what you become but remember the better choice is almost always harder, costlier and more challenging. So, choose it wisely. Focus on solutions, not on problems. Look for opportunities to do great work instead of waiting and doing nothing. Have a positive attitude instead of negative.

#7. Power of 'Enough is enough'

Are you satisfied with the amount of success you have had in your life so far? Don't you think you are a lot more capable than what you have achieved in your life so far? Just say no more mediocracy, it's time to go and fly high. Say no more excuses, it's time to raise the bar and set high standards. Stand tall and say 'Enough is enough' it's time to be a genius. Yes, 'The Genius You' has been unleashed!

You don't need expensive running shoes, you need to get out and run. You don't need more time, you need to use it better to make the most of it. You don't need more resources, you need to better use the resources that you already have. You don't need more opportunities, you need to take advantage of the ones in front of you. If you want to be genius, it's not about what looks good or seems easier, it's about doing what's necessary.

Everyone wants to go to heaven but nobody wants to die. Everyone wants to be known as an extraordinary performer but nobody wants to give what it takes to be a peak-performer. Everyone wants success but nobody is ready to pay the price.

What about you? Are you ready to have a radical shift in your life? If yes, start acting now. I wish you a wonderful life ahead! Be a genius, the whole world is waiting for you to show what you are capable of. Unleash the genius within you and let your new life start now!

My Genius Roadmap

My Empowering Statement:

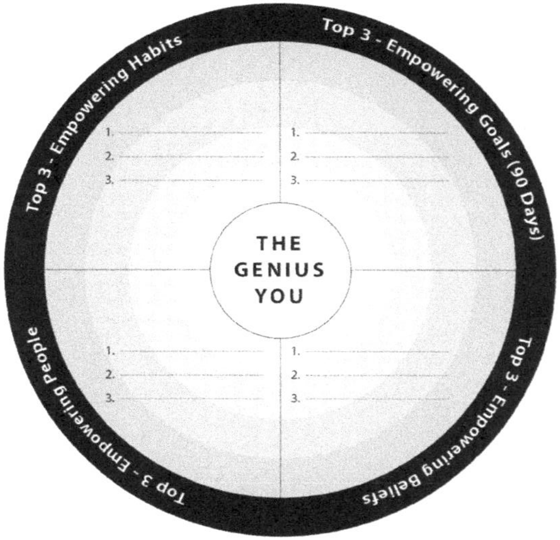

1. My thinking pattern is ______.
   (sustain/opportunistic)
2. I have ______ mindset.
   (growth/fixed)
3. I'm in ______ state most of the time.
   (resourceful/unresourceful)
4. I ______ 11 maxims.
   (follow/don't follow)
5. I ______ consistent action.
   (take/don't take)

Top 3 - Five Years Goals

1. ______
2. ______
3. ______